Earn CME credits while you

Up to 75 *AMA PRA Category 1 Credits*™ ava........ ... ...
MedStudy 2013 Internal Medicine Board-Style Questions & Answers

Release Date: October 15, 2012   Expiration Date: October 15, 2015

Learning Objectives

As a result of participation in this activity, learners will be able to:

- Integrate and demonstrate increased overall knowledge of Internal Medicine

- Identify and remedy areas of weakness (gaps) in knowledge and clinical competencies

- Describe the clinical manifestations and treatments of diseases encountered in Internal Medicine and effectively narrow the differential diagnosis list by utilizing the most appropriate medical studies

- Apply the competence and confidence gained through participation in this activity to both a successful Board exam-taking experience and daily practice

Target Audience

Physicians seeking to assess, expand, and/or reinforce their knowledge and decision-making strategies in the broad fields of Internal Medicine as they prepare for their American Board of Internal Medicine (ABIM) Certification and Maintenance of Certification (MoC) Board exams.

Learner Participation

The content of this self-study CME activity is designed to help learners assess their own key knowledge and clinical competencies with evidence-based standards of care, which are reflected on the Board exams. Use the multiple-choice, question-answer content as a self-testing exercise, attempting to answer questions as though they are part of an actual Board exam. Compare your selected answers against the answers given as "correct" in the Answer Book to assess your level of knowledge and recall of pertinent medical facts and clinical decision-making. Review your results to see your relative strengths and weaknesses by topic areas. Repeat the self-testing process as often as necessary to improve your knowledge and proficiency and ultimately to ensure your mastery of the material.

Continuing Medical Education

MedStudy is accredited by the Accreditation Council for Continuing Medical Education (ACCME) to provide continuing medical education for physicians.

MedStudy designates this enduring material for a maximum of **75** *AMA PRA Category 1 Credits*™. Physicians should claim only the credit commensurate with the extent of their participation in the activity.

This credit may be submitted to the American Osteopathic Association (AOA) for category 2 credit. All other health care professionals completing this continuing education activity will be issued a certificate of participation.

How to Apply for CME Credit

Please note: CME credit is available **only** to the original purchaser of this product, and issuance of CME credit is subject to verification of product ownership. CME credits for the 2013 Internal Medicine Q&As will be available until October 15, 2015. (1 hour = 1 CME credit)

1. Study the material as often as necessary in order to understand and master the content.
2. Go to www.MedStudy.com and click on CME in the menu bar.
3. In the MedStudy CME Program table, find the link: <u>Download 2013 IM Q&As CME Application</u>.
4. Once you have downloaded the application, follow the instructions for completing the CME credit application, post-test, and product evaluation.

Note: For any questions, please email us at cme@medstudy.com or call 1-800-841-0547, ext. 3.

Author/Editor:

J. Thomas Cross, Jr., MD, MPH, FACP
Director of Medical Education
MedStudy Corporation
Colorado Springs, Colorado

Contributors:

Seth Mark Berney, MD *
Professor of Medicine
Chief, Section of Rheumatology
Director, Center of Excellence for Arthritis and
Rheumatology
Louisiana State University Health Sciences Center
Shreveport, Louisiana

Ronea Harris-Stith, MD, FAAD
Medical Director
Refined Dermatology Resources, PC
Charlotte, North Carolina

Steve Karceski, MD *
Associate Clinical Professor of Neurology
Director of Clinical Trials
Cornell Comprehensive Epilepsy Center
Weill Cornell Medical College
Cornell University
New York, New York

Vinay Maheshwari, MD, FCCP
Medical Director, Respiratory Therapy
Pulmonary, Critical Care and Sleep Medicine
Pulmonary Associates, PA
Christiana Care Health Systems
Wilmington, Delaware

Sriram Narsipur, MD, FASN
Associate Professor of Medicine and Pediatrics
Nephrology Division
SUNY Upstate Medical University
Syracuse, New York

Douglas Paauw, MD, MACP
Professor of Medicine
Rathmann Family Foundation Endowed Chair
in Patient-Centered Clinical Education
Head, Section of GIM, Department of Medicine
University of Washington School of Medicine
Seattle, Washington

Kimberly Salkey, MD
Assistant Professor
Department of Dermatology
Eastern Virginia Medical School
Norfolk, Virginia

Janet Schlechte, MD, FACP
Professor of Medicine
Division of Endocrinology and Metabolism
Department of Internal Medicine
University of Iowa
Iowa City, Iowa

Candace L. Walkley, MD
Associate Director of Medical Education
MedStudy Corporation
Colorado Springs, Colorado

N.S. Teddy Winstead, MD, MSPH, FACP *
Director, Gastroenterology Clinical Research
Department of Gastroenterology and Hepatology
Ochsner Clinic
New Orleans, Louisiana

Note: Those contributors with an asterisk (*) after their names have disclosed relationships with entities producing, marketing, re-selling, or distributing health care goods or services consumed by, or used on, patients (see next page). All others have documented they have **no** relationships with such entities.

MedStudy Disclosure Policy

It is the policy of MedStudy to ensure balance, independence, objectivity, and scientific rigor in all of its educational activities. In keeping with all policies of MedStudy and the Accreditation Council for Continuing Medical Education (ACCME), any contributor to a MedStudy CME activity is required to disclose all relevant relationships with any entity producing, marketing, re-selling, or distributing health care goods or services consumed by, or used on, patients. Failure to do so precludes acceptance by MedStudy of any material by that individual. All contributors are also required to submit a signed Good Practices Agreement affirming that their contribution is based upon currently available, scientifically rigorous data; that it is free from commercial bias; and that any clinical practice and patient care recommendations offered are based on the best available evidence for these specialties and subspecialties. All content is carefully reviewed by MedStudy's CME Physicians Oversight Council, as well as on-staff copyreaders, and any perceived issues or conflicts are resolved prior to publication of an enduring product or the start of a live activity.

Contributor Disclosures

The following contributors have openly indicated affiliation with commercial entities.

Seth Mark Berney, MD
Grant/Research: Biogen Idec, Genentech, MedImmune, Roche
Major Stockholder: Pfizer

Steve Karceski, MD
Grant/Research: Cyberonics
Speakers' Bureau: Cyberonics, UCB

N.S. Teddy Winstead, MD, MSPH, FACP
Grant/Research: Janssen, UCB
Speakers' Bureau: Janssen, UCB

MedStudy Disclosure

MedStudy Corporation, including all of its employees, has **no** financial interest, arrangement or affiliation with any commercial entity producing, marketing, re-selling, or distributing health care goods or services consumed by, or used on, patients. Furthermore, MedStudy complies with the AMA Council on Ethical and Judicial Affairs (CEJA) opinions that address the ethical obligations that underpin physician participation in CME: 8.061, "Gifts to physicians from industry," and 9.011, "Ethical issues in CME."

For Further Study

MedStudy Internal Medicine Review Core Curriculum, 15th Edition.
MedStudy Corporation, Colorado Springs, CO, 2013.

MedStudy Internal Medicine Core Scripts®, 2013–2014 Edition (flash cards).
MedStudy Corporation, Colorado Springs, CO, 2013.

MedStudy 2013 or 2014 Video Board Review of Internal Medicine.
MedStudy Corporation, Colorado Springs, CO. 2013 and 2014.

MedStudy 2013 or 2014 Recertification Video Board Review of Internal Medicine.
MedStudy Corporation, Colorado Springs, CO. 2013 and 2014.

Harrison's Principles of Internal Medicine, 18th Edition.
Dan L. Longo, Anthony S. Fauci, Dennis L. Kasper, Stephen L. Hauser, J. Larry Jameson, and Joseph Loscalzo (eds).
McGraw-Hill Medical, 2012.

Cecil Medicine, 24th Edition. Lee Goldman, MD, and Andrew I. Schafer, MD. Saunders Elsevier, 2012.

Web-based:
National Guideline Clearinghouse: http://www.ahrq.gov/
American College of Physicians Guidelines: www.acponline.org/clinical_information/guidelines

MedStudy®

Internal Medicine Board-Style Questions & Answers

2013

QUESTIONS

J. Thomas Cross, Jr., MD, MPH, FACP

TABLE OF CONTENTS

Disclaimers

Important: These Q&A books are meant to be used as an adjunct to the MedStudy Internal Medicine Review Core Curriculum. The ABIM exams cover a vast realm of diagnostic and treatment knowledge. Board-simulation exercise such as these self-testing Q&As are valuable tools, but these alone are not adequate preparation for a Board exam. Be sure you use a comprehensive IM review resource in addition to these Q&As for adequate exam preparation.

Content: The primary purpose of this activity is educational. Medicine and accepted standards of care are constantly changing. We at MedStudy do our best to review and include in this activity accurate discussions of the standards of care, methods of diagnosis, and selection of treatments. However, the authors/presenters, editors, advisors, and publisher—and all other parties involved with the preparation of this work—disclaim any guarantee that the information contained in this activity and its associated materials is in every respect accurate or complete. MedStudy further disclaims any and all liability for damages and claims that may result from the use of information or viewpoints presented. We recommend you confirm the information contained in this activity and in any other educational material with current sources of medical knowledge whenever considering actual clinical presentations or treating patients.

ABIM: For over 20 years, MedStudy has excelled in determining and teaching what a clinically competent Internal Medicine physician should know. The American Board of Internal Medicine (ABIM) tests this exact same pool of knowledge. MedStudy's expertise, demonstrated by the superb pass rate of those who use it in their studies, is in the actual "teaching" of this knowledge in a clear, learner-friendly manner that results in a stronger knowledge base, improved clinical skills, and better Board results. Although what we teach is in sync with what the Boards test, MedStudy has no affiliation with the ABIM, and our authors, editors, and reviewers have no access to ABIM exam content. Our material is developed as original work by MedStudy physician authors, with additional input from expert contributors, based on their extensive backgrounds in professional medical education. This content is designed to include subject matter typically tested in certification and recertification exams as outlined in the ABIM's publicly available exam blueprints but makes no use of, and divulges no details of, ABIM's proprietary exam content.

A note on editorial style: MedStudy uses a standardized approach to the naming of diseases. The previous method of naming was to use the possessive form that adds " 's " to the names of diseases and disorders, such as Lou Gehrig's disease, Klinefelter's syndrome, and others. In MedStudy material, you will see the non-possessive form when the proper name is followed by a common noun; e.g., "This patient would warrant workup for Crohn disease." Exceptions to the possessive form include Bell's palsy and Still's murmur. Possessive form will be used, however, when an entity is referred to solely by its proper name without a following common noun; e.g., "The symptoms are classic for Crohn's." *The AMA Manual of Style*, *JAMA*, and *Scientific Style and Format* are among the publications that promote and use the non-possessive form.

MEDSTUDY
1455 Quail Lake Loop
Colorado Springs, CO 80906
(800) 841-0547
www.medstudy.com

About the questions and answers in this learning activity

The questions, answers, and explanations in this learning activity are developed by the author, based on his own background of 21 years in professional medical education and his ongoing consultation with many subspecialty experts from around the country. Dr. Cross is also an author/editor for MedStudy's Internal Medicine Review Core Curriculum and a teacher at MedStudy's live Internal Medicine Certification and Recertification Board Review courses. He has previously been an associate professor in the Departments of Internal Medicine and Pediatrics at Louisiana State University Health Sciences Center and is a past president of the National Internal Medicine/Pediatrics Program Directors' Association. Dr. Cross is Board Certified in Internal Medicine, Pediatrics, and in both Adult and Pediatric Infectious Disease (ID).

Knowing the importance that the IM Boards place on established standards of care, having researched recent and pertinent practice guidelines, and having reviewed the publicly available ABIM Board exam blueprints, Dr. Cross is well aware of the areas of knowledge most likely to be tested on today's Board exams. As a result, you will find that the percentage of questions by topic in this activity mirrors the Board template. You will find questions of varying length here. The very short ones are designed to nail home an important point you need to know and remember for your Boards. The lengthier questions help you integrate content on a subject with additional clinical information to better simulate a real-life patient scenario.

This helps you recognize disease states and associated treatment, which is a skill heavily tested on Board exams. Some selected patient case scenarios may appear more than once, or with only slight variations, with the associated questions addressing different diagnoses and treatment aspects of the case. This is in keeping with the approach Board questions take in limiting patient case assessments to one key testing point.

In short, this Q&A material is designed to impart not only relevant knowledge for IM Board exams but also challenge your skills in interpretation and intervention, which is what Board exams attempt to assess. Which is why we call these, appropriately, "Board-style" questions and answers.

There is a popular misconception that members of organizations perceived to be associated with medical boards write Board exam questions; e.g., ACP/MKSAP with the American Board of Internal Medicine or AAP/PREP with the American Board of Pediatrics. Not only is this not true, it is actually forbidden for anyone to write formal Board exam questions if they work for a company or organization in the business of producing Board preparation materials. This would compromise the integrity of the examining process.

MedStudy is proud to be able to bring you Board-style questions and answers of the highest quality—to offer you education that is relevant in a format that reinforces your knowledge to prepare you well for whatever challenge the ABIM Board exam presents you. One final note: Even the best question-and-answer exercise by itself is not an adequate preparation for a Board exam. These Q&As should be used as an adjunct to a comprehensive Board review course (such as MedStudy's Internal Medicine Review Core Curriculum). The Boards cover a vast realm of information that Board simulation Q&As alone cannot encompass.

GASTROENTEROLOGY

1.

A 45-year-old man undergoes screening colonoscopy because of a family history of colorectal cancer (his father at age 48). The preparation is adequate, and the endoscopist reaches the cecum. A single, 8-mm polyp is removed, and the pathology report shows hyperplastic tissue.

At what age should he undergo another colonoscopy?

A. 50
B. 55
C. 48
D. 46

2.

An 80-year-old African-American man with a history of blood transfusions in 1989 after a motor vehicle accident is noted to have an ALT of 300 while on lipid-lowering therapy. He denies any complaints of icteric illness, or any family history of liver disease. His workup is remarkable for a +hepatitis C antibody with a viral load of 1.6 million IU/mL. His genotype is 1a. An ultrasound of the liver shows a completely normal liver echotexture with a few small 3- to 4-mm gallstones. His bilirubin and alkaline phosphatase are normal.

The next appropriate step would be which of the following?

A. Refer for cholecystectomy.
B. Start peginterferon and ribavirin only.
C. Refer for liver biopsy.
D. Observation only.
E. Stop atorvastatin.

3.

A 50-year-old African-American woman presents to GI clinic because of gas, bloating, and diarrhea anytime she drinks milk or eats cheese or ice cream. Symptoms are slightly better when taking an over-the-counter lactase enzyme preparation. Her mother has the same problem. She had a normal colonoscopy last year for colorectal cancer screening. The endoscopist did random colon biopsies that were normal.

The next appropriate step is which of the following?

A. Celiac antibodies
B. Empiric treatment with metronidazole 250 mg PO tid x 10 d
C. Repeat colonoscopy with random biopsies
D. Lactose avoidance
E. Small bowel x-ray to rule out Crohn disease

4.

A 40-year-old obese woman presents with heartburn. She also has intermittent dysphagia to solids and liquids, so she undergoes an EGD that shows significant (Stage III) erosive esophagitis. She is started on a PPI. She continues on the PPI for 12 weeks with marked improvement of symptoms. She has a trial off the PPI, and symptoms return within several weeks. Restarting the PPI provides relief. She returns to clinic inquiring as to how long she should take this medicine because she has seen stories on the nightly news about fracture risk. She has no family history of osteoporosis or increased risk of fractures.

In addition to making sure she takes in adequate calcium and vitamin D, you tell her to continue her PPI for how long?

A. 3 weeks
B. 3 months
C. 3 years
D. Forever

5.

You are moonlighting in the ER when a 30-year-old presents with melena, hematemesis (bright red blood), and orthostasis. She does not drink; she has no stigmata of chronic liver disease; she does not have any risk factors. She has been taking ibuprofen 800 mg tid for a sore ankle. Her initial blood pressure is 60/40; pulse is 113 beats per minute; and her initial hematocrit is 14.

Which of the following is the next most appropriate step in management?

A. Call for GI consult and emergent upper endoscopy
B. IV normal saline bolus, type and crossmatch, emergent upper endoscopy
C. IV normal saline bolus, type and crossmatch
D. IV D5W and emergent upper endoscopy

6.

What is the observed mortality benefit from screening colonoscopy due to?

A. Removal of adenomas
B. Detection of bacterial overgrowth
C. Removal of hyperplastic polyps
D. Detection of incident cancers

7.

A 40-year-old man undergoes endoscopy for heartburn and dysphagia. At endoscopy, he is found to have 3 small duodenal ulcers and LA class D reflux esophagitis. He is placed on esomeprazole. Because of this presentation, he undergoes fasting serum gastrin testing. His gastrin level is 600 pg/dL (upper limit normal is 110 pg/dL). He returns to your clinic.

What do you tell him about his gastrin elevation?

    A. It is likely that he has gastrinoma.
    B. It is likely that he has atrophic gastritis.
    C. It is likely from taking esomeprazole.
    D. It is likely from primary G-cell hyperplasia.

8.

A 32-year-old white female is referred to you for anemia. She has had Crohn disease for 15 years and has had one surgery, but she doesn't remember the details. She is currently on no medications. She has diarrhea, moving her bowels about 8 times per day. Once or twice a month she also has postprandial vomiting. Her Hct is 30%, and her MCV is 102.

Her Crohn disease is likely which of the following?

    A. Inactive, in the terminal ileum
    B. Active, in the terminal ileum
    C. Active, gastroduodenal
    D. Inactive, gastroduodenal

9.

An 89-year-old with congestive heart failure, pulmonary hypertension, and emphysema is referred to you because of iron deficiency. Her Hct is 30; her ferritin is 1; and her MCV is 70. These values are stable, and 2 years ago she had an EGD and colonoscopy, both of which were normal. Her stool is heme negative and brown. She never has had melena or hematochezia.

You recommend which of the following?

    A. Do nothing except oral iron and prn transfusions.
    B. CT of the abdomen.
    C. EGD, colonoscopy, and videocapsule endoscopy.
    D. CT angiography.

10.

A 21-year-old man is referred for abdominal pain for 5 years. He has had a workup from an outside gastroenterologist including CT, retroperitoneal Doppler, EGD and colonoscopy (both with biopsies), and videocapsule endoscopy.

What is the next _most_ appropriate step?

    A. Questioning about sexual and physical abuse
    B. Serum gastrin level
    C. Repeat entire workup
    D. Celiac disease serology

11.

A 19-year-old female who has recently been diagnosed with celiac disease presents to your clinic to establish care. During the visit, she seeks your advice concerning the anticipated course of her celiac disease.

Which of the following is true regarding her condition?

    A. Pancrease supplements will improve the malabsorption effects.
    B. She is at increased risk for Addison disease and lymphomas.
    C. Rye or barley products should replace wheat products.
    D. Dapsone therapy will reduce her gastrointestinal complaints.

12.

A 22-year-old female presents with a pruritic rash that recurrently develops blisters over the elbows, knees, and back. Symptomatic interventions and topical steroids have had no effect. Due to the intensity of symptoms, the patient is referred for dermatologic evaluation where direct immunofluorescence of a biopsy specimen is diagnostic for dermatitis herpetiformis.

This condition is <u>most</u> strongly associated with which of the following pathologies?

    A. Zinc deficiency
    B. Peutz-Jeghers syndrome
    C. Gluten sensitivity
    D. Crohn disease

13.

A 32-year-old woman presents to your office with a complaint of abdominal pain. She describes generalized pain that occurs 4–5 times per month since she was a teenager. She notes that her stools often become loose after she notices the pain, but that it improves after she defecates. She reports she occasionally sees blood in her stool with intense straining during a bowel movement. She denies fever, nausea, vomiting, or weight loss. Her past medical history is significant for generalized anxiety for which she takes citalopram.

Physical exam is notable for mild tenderness to palpation in the LLQ without rebound or guarding. Digital rectal exam demonstrates normal tone without palpable mass. The remainder of the exam is normal.

Which of the following is the next best step in the management of this patient?

    A. Tissue transglutaminase antibody testing
    B. Fecal occult blood testing
    C. CT of the abdomen
    D. Begin therapy with loperamide
    E. Begin therapy with amitriptyline

14.

A 26-year-old woman presents to your office for abdominal pain. She reports that she has episodes of crampy abdominal pain with a sensation of feeling bloated 2 times a week associated with constipation for the last 8 years. She reports that her pain improves after defecation. She denies fever, rectal bleeding, or weight loss. She notes that she recently lost her job. She feels anxious because she already had to cancel one job interview due to abdominal pain and feels that this has caused her symptoms to worsen. She reports taking over-the-counter psyllium to try to improve her constipation without success. Her past medical history is otherwise unremarkable, and she currently takes no medications.

Physical exam reveals a thin woman in no acute distress. Abdominal exam is notable for palpable bowel loop in the left lower quadrant with mild tenderness without rebound or guarding. The remainder of the physical exam is normal. Fecal occult blood testing is negative.

Which of the following is the next best step in the management of this patient?

    A. Amitriptyline
    B. Citalopram
    C. Dicyclomine
    D. Polyethylene glycol 3350
    E. Senna

15.

A 28-year-old man presents to your office with a complaint of abdominal pain. He reports a history of generalized crampy pain occurring several times per week that has gone on for several years. He reports that he occasionally has diarrhea that accompanies the pain. Further questioning elicits that he has had mild fatigue that has rarely interfered with his daily activities. He reports that he participated in a fast with his co-workers in attempt to "cleanse" himself by abstaining from solid foods for 2 weeks. He stated that his symptoms resolved completely but subsequently returned after resuming his regular diet. His physical examination is otherwise unremarkable. You obtain the following laboratory studies:

WBC 9.2/uL (4.0–10 x 10^9/L)
Hgb 13.8 g/dL (14–17g/dL)
Hct 39.5% (41–51%)
Plt 298/uL (150–350 x 10^9/L)
MCV 75 fL (80–100 fL)
Ferritin 12 ng/mL (15–200 ng/mL)
TIBC 385 ug/dL (250–460 ug/dL)
Serum Iron 44 ug/dL (60–160 ug/dL)
Fecal occult blood testing – Negative
Anti-tissue Transglutaminase Antibody – Positive

What is the next best step in the management of this patient?

    A. Endomysial antibody testing
    B. Upper EGD with small bowel biopsy
    C. Iron replacement therapy
    D. Initiation of gluten-free diet
    E. Colonoscopy

16.

A 46-year-old male patient presents to the clinic with complaints of repeated vomiting. Of greatest concern to the patient is the presence of blood in the emesis.

Which of the following is <u>most</u> specific for peptic ulcer disease as the source for the vomited blood?

    A. Bright red blood following an emesis episode
    B. Mucoid emesis with streaks of blood
    C. Large volumes of regurgitated bright blood
    D. Specks of blood with black particulate emesis

17.

A 66-year-old male is seen in the clinic after referral from his dentist due to the recent development of halitosis. His dental exam was unremarkable. The patient states that he has experienced increasing difficulty swallowing that worsens as he progresses through a meal. He also relates that he regurgitates food that appears undigested hours after a meal. He has lost 5 pounds over the preceding 6 months.

A barium swallow reveals a 6-cm posterior pouch in the upper esophagus. The mucosa appears smooth, and the remainder of the exam is reported as normal.

Which of the following statements is true regarding this patient?

    A. Effectiveness of medications may be reduced in this condition.
    B. Institution of a motility agent will help relieve symptoms.
    C. Direct endoscopic examination is required.
    D. Esophageal manometry will aid in treatment decisions.

18.

A 62-year-old female presents to the emergency department with complaints of acute abdominal pain. The pain started during the previous night with periumbilical discomfort and nausea. Over the next 16 hours, the pain localized over the left lower abdominal quadrant. She has experienced a feverish feeling and gassiness but has not been able to have a bowel movement. Her past history is remarkable for a total hysterectomy with bilateral ovary removal 10 years previously. She has a history of diverticulosis.

On physical examination, the patient is in moderate distress with a temperature of 100.2° F (37.9° C). Bowel sounds are present but hypoactive. The patient has significant guarding with tenderness in the left lower abdomen about 3 cm above the inguinal ligament. No rebound is noted. There is nonspecific CVA tenderness.

Which of the following is the <u>most</u> appropriate diagnostic test at this time?

    A. 3 views of the abdomen
    B. CT scan of the abdomen
    C. Barium enema
    D. Colonoscopy

19.

A 45-year-old female is seen in your clinic complaining of swall[...]
complaints of intermittent regurgitation for several years but has [...]
episodes. When she vomits, the emesis consists of nonbilious flu[...]
any blood or significant pain. She recently became more concer[...]
a meal eaten several days previously, despite having eaten sever[...]

The physical exam is most remarkable for significant halitosis. [...]
CBC and electrolytes are within normal limits.

Which of the following is the most likely diagnosis?

A. Mallory-Weiss tear
B. Plummer-Vinson syndrome
C. Zenker diverticulum
D. Achalasia

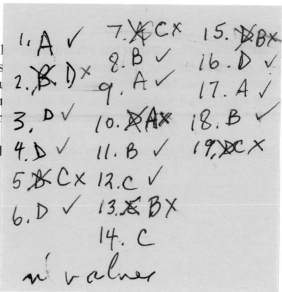

20.

A 27-year-old male presents to the clinic with abdominal cramping and bloody diarrhea. He has recently returned from international travel as a Peace Corps worker.

Which of the following would be the most likely agent to present with grossly bloody diarrhea?

A. *Entamoeba histolytica*
B. *Vibrio cholerae*
C. Norovirus
D. *Bacillus cereus*
E. *Staphylococcus aureus*

21.

A 39-year-old female with an extended history of alcoholism, hepatitis B infection, cirrhosis, and ascites presents to the emergency department with complaints of abdominal tenderness and fever. The pain started 10–12 hours previously and was initially periumbilical. Nausea developed shortly following the onset of pain. Over the next several hours, the pain became more severe and localized in the right lower abdomen. She has vomited several times and feels constipated but has not been able to pass stool.

On examination, the patient is in obvious distress. Her temperature is 101.8° F (38.8° C). Her abdominal exam is remarkable for significant ascites, hyperactive bowel sounds, and abdominal tenderness. The greatest discomfort is in the right lower quadrant, and there is rebound on deep palpation in that area.

WBC is elevated at $16.5 \times 10^3/mm^3$ with a significant left shift.

In addition to analgesia, which of the following is the **most** important intervention at this time?

A. Diagnostic and therapeutic peritoneal tap
B. Spiral CT of the abdomen
C. GI referral for colonoscopy
D. Urgent evaluation for TIPS procedure
E. Surgical exploration of the abdomen

22.

A 56-year-old male is diagnosed with pancreatic cancer located in the head of the pancreas and impinging on the common duct. Following consultation with oncology and surgery, a Whipple procedure (resection of the head of the pancreas with reanastomoses of the pancreatic and biliary tract) is performed.

Following the procedure, which of the following feeding methods offers the best advantage?

A. Nasogastric (NG) tube gavage feedings
B. Percutaneous gastric (PEG) tube feedings
C. Jejunal tube (J-tube) feedings
D. Peripheral nutrition through a PICC line

23.

A 54-year-old male presents as a new patient for refills of his omeprazole prescription. He has been taking this medication for 3 years with very good control of his symptoms. He reports that an upper GI series 3 years ago demonstrated a sliding hiatal hernia. He is otherwise well with no social risk factors.

Of the following, the **most serious consequence of a persistent hiatal hernia is:**

A. Esophageal cancer
B. Stomach cancer
C. Aspiration pneumonia
D. Pernicious anemia

24.

During the long-term treatment of a 26-year-old male with ulcerative colitis, the patient requires intermittent pulses of glucocorticosteroids to gain symptomatic control.

Which of the following is true regarding the use of corticosteroids in the treatment of ulcerative colitis?

A. Rectal steroids avoid adrenal suppressive effects.
B. Corticosteroids are a principal agent to maintain remissions.
C. Risk of avascular necrosis is increased with steroid usage.
D. Active steroid use decreases the risk of malignant degeneration.

25.

A 65-year-old female presents to the clinic with diarrhea that has been present for the last 7 days. The stool is watery and no blood has been noted. She is not toxic appearing, and her WBC is normal. She does not have fever. Her recent history is important for a skin abscess that was treated with a 10-day course of antibiotics 5 weeks ago.

Stool studies reveal normal flora on cultures with no significant blood or fecal leukocytes noted. Evaluation for *C. difficile* toxin is positive.

Which of the following is the <u>most</u> appropriate intervention at this time?

    A. Admit for intravenous vancomycin.
    B. Institute a course of oral metronidazole.
    C. Recommend over-the-counter loperamide.
    D. Prescribe a course of oral clindamycin.

26.

Following an evaluation for unexpected hepatic dysfunction, a patient in your practice is diagnosed with hemochromatosis.

Which of the following is the <u>most</u> effective therapy for hemochromatosis?

    A. Repetitive phlebotomy
    B. Intravenous deferoxamine
    C. Exchange transfusion
    D. Interferon therapy

27.

You are asked to follow up with a 47-year-old female who was recently hospitalized for pancreatitis associated with a biliary stone. The stone passed spontaneously, and the patient was treated with analgesics and IV fluids until she was able to resume oral intake. She was doing well until earlier this morning when she experienced increasing abdominal pain and feverishness. The patient continues with a temperature of 102.8° F (39.3° C). CBC revealed WBC of $18.9 \times 10^3/mm^3$. An urgent CT scan of the abdomen was ordered and shows evidence of early pancreatic necrosis.

The <u>most</u> important intervention at this time would be:

    A. Blood cultures and broad-spectrum antibiotics
    B. CT-guided aspiration of the pancreatic necrotic tissue
    C. Endoscopic retrograde cholangiopancreatography (ERCP)
    D. Emergent surgical consult

28.

A 35-year-old female presents to the clinic with a one-month history of a small amount of bright red blood following bowel movements. There is a mild amount of discomfort associated with the bleeding. Her periods have been normal, and she expresses no other complaints.

Rectal examination is impressive for a moderately enlarged posterior external hemorrhoid. Digital rectal exam is unremarkable, and guaiac testing is weakly positive. CBC reveals borderline low hematocrit/hemoglobin levels.

Which of the following is the <u>most</u> appropriate intervention at this time?

    A. Institute iron supplements and recheck hemoglobin in 3 months.
    B. Recommend an increase in dietary fiber and over-the-counter hemorrhoid cream.
    C. Refer to surgery for sigmoidoscopy and hemorrhoidal banding.
    D. Refer the patient for gastroenterology for colonoscopy.

29.

A 27-year-old male presents to the emergency department with complaints of rectal pain that has been progressing over the last 24 hours. He states he has been feverish with some nausea and has pain that is much worse with defecation.

On physical examination, his temperature is 101.8° F (38.8° C). Bowel sounds are present and the abdomen is soft. On examination of the rectum, a 1.3-cm pustule is noted at the anal verge with surrounding erythema and tenderness. Digital rectal exam is not possible due to the exquisite tenderness.

Based on this information, which of the following is the <u>most</u> important intervention for this patient?

    A. Diagnostic sigmoidoscopy
    B. Incision and drainage of the pustule
    C. Surgical exploration and debridement
    D. Admission for IV antibiotics

30.

A 43-year-old man presents to your clinic with concerns over long-term problems with diarrhea. He has experienced frequent loose stools for nearly two years. Of more concern to the patient is the fact that the stools are now associated with bloating and episodes of explosive diarrhea, and the associated smell is becoming almost unbearable. Other than the abdominal complaints, he has experienced some intermittent joint aching that seems to move from joint to joint and responds to occasional NSAIDs.

His abdominal exam reveals some abdominal distention but no marked tenderness and no abnormal masses.

Initial stool studies are remarkable for large quantities of fecal fat and a moderate amount of fecal leukocytes. Stool culture and examination for ova and parasites are negative. Along with additional laboratory studies, HIV testing is also negative.

Subsequent evaluation included small bowel biopsy, which demonstrated PAS (+) macrophages.

Appropriate therapy for this condition would be:

    A. Strict avoidance of gluten-containing foods
    B. Antibiotic therapy
    C. Pancreatic supplements and avoidance of long chain fats
    D. Therapy with high-dose oral steroids

31.

You are asked to consult with a 31-year-old man for the evaluation of jaundice. Two days ago, he underwent operative repair of a right medial meniscus tear, and yesterday the surgeon noted the patient became yellow. The patient is asymptomatic and has never had chronic health problems. He takes no medications except Percocet® for postoperative pain, and he has had no known exposures or travel outside the U.S. He is up-to-date with immunizations. He drinks 2–3 beers a week. He does not use any illicit drugs.

ROS: He recalls similar eye discoloration after "the flu" 2 years ago.

Physical exam is normal except for scleral icterus and jaundice, and surgical dressings on the right knee.

Laboratory results:

HBsAg:	Negative
Anti-HBs antibody:	Positive
Anti-HBc (IgM):	Negative
HAV ab:	Negative
AST:	40 U/L
ALT:	36 U/L
Alk Phos:	110 U/L
Bili: (T)	3.2 mg/dL
Bili: (D)	0.4 mg/dL

Complete blood count and basic metabolic panel are normal. Urinalysis is negative.

What is the <u>most</u> appropriate next step in patient care?

    A. Right upper-quadrant ultrasound
    B. Liver biopsy
    C. Initiation of pegylated interferon plus ribavirin
    D. Endoscopic retrograde cholangiopancreatography
    E. Reassurance

32.

A 34-year-old woman presents with a 3-year history of rectal bleeding, abdominal pain, and weight loss. Colonoscopy with biopsy is performed; histology shows acute and chronic mucosal inflammation, crypt distortion with forked glands, and crypt atrophy. You begin sulfasalazine 4 gm daily.

Three weeks later, she feels much better, and bleeding has stopped. However, on routine follow-up labs, the following is noted:

Laboratory results:

		Normals
WBC:	11,500	3,500–10,000 cells/mm^3
WBC differential:	Normal	
ALT:	70	0–35 U/L
AST:	65	0–35 U/L
Alk Phos:	428	36–92 U/L
Total bilirubin:	1.4	0.3–1.2 mg/dL
Albumin:	3.1	3.5–5.5 g/dL
Total protein:	6.0	6.0–7.8 g/dL
BMP:	Normal	
PT:	11.0	11–13 seconds
PTT:	20.8	25–25 seconds
Urinalysis:	Normal	

RUQ ultrasound is performed; no stones or CBD dilatation are seen.

Which of the following findings is <u>most</u> likely to be present?

    A. Multifocal stricturing and dilation of intrahepatic bile ducts on cholangiography
    B. Elevated antimitochondrial antibodies and ANA; bridging fibrosis on liver biopsy
    C. HBsAg positive, anti-HBe positive, eventual resolution of liver enzymes
    D. Multiple areas of increased uptake on three-phase bone scan
    E. A large, heterogeneous hepatic mass on contrast CT of the liver

33.

A 76-year-old man presents with new-onset dysphagia. He describes his dysphagia for solids and liquids for about the past 4 weeks. He has no prior history of dysphagia. He also describes nocturnal regurgitation of sour food.

Past Medical History: Significant for COPD from long-standing tobacco use (60-pack-years).

Review of Systems: He has stable dyspnea on exertion and a chronic cough, but has recently developed a nocturnal cough. He has lost 20 pounds over the last month. He denies chest pain.

Physical Exam: RR 18 bpm
Mild cachexia
Barrel-shaped chest with an increased expiratory phase; scattered bilateral wheezes.
The abdomen is normal.

Barium swallow: Dilated esophagus with bird beak narrowing of the distal esophagus.

Which of the following is the <u>most</u> appropriate next step in diagnosis?

    A. Esophageal motility.
    B. Esophagogastroduodenoscopy (EGD).
    C. Refer to surgery for laparoscopic myotomy.
    D. Start empiric omeprazole and reevaluate in 4 weeks.
    E. Schedule Botox$^{®}$ injection.

34.

A 25-year-old male complains of intermittent dysphagia for solids and liquids. In fact, most episodes have occurred for cold liquids about twice a month. Typically, the dysphagia has occurred while the patient is at work. He denies any heartburn or regurgitation.

Past Medical History: Healthy.
Social History: Negative for cigarettes and alcohol. He has an irregular diet with long hours at his job as a junior lawyer at a large law firm.
Physical Exam: Normal.
Barium Swallow:

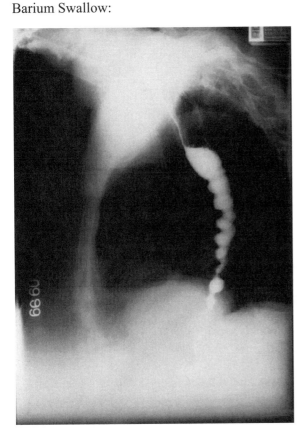

Which of the following is definitely <u>not</u> indicated?

    A. Twice daily calcium channel antagonist
    B. Sildenafil once daily
    C. Amitriptyline 50 mg before bed
    D. Schedule esophagogastroduodenoscopy (EGD)
    E. Reassurance

35.

A 28-year-old Hispanic male complains of belching and abdominal fullness after meals. He denies ever having significant abdominal pain. The symptoms increase after certain foods, large meals, and carbonated beverages; although sometimes he reports that the ingestion of small meals will actually help his symptoms. These symptoms are present 2–3 days out of each week. The symptoms have never awakened him from sleep. He denies any heartburn, dysphagia, and use of NSAIDs. He is a recent immigrant from Mexico.

Past Medical History:	Normal
Physical Exam:	Normal
Social History:	Negative for tobacco or alcohol
Review of Systems:	No weight loss, melena, or change in bowel habits
Complete blood count:	Normal

Which of the following is the <u>most</u> appropriate next step in patient care?

    A. Upper GI series
    B. Esophagogastroduodenoscopy (EGD)
    C. Abdominal CT scan
    D. *H. pylori* ELISA with treatment if positive
    E. Gallbladder ultrasound

36.

A 52-year-old male has just returned from a Colorado camping trip with his college friends. He mentions how great the hiking was and how wonderful the water from the pristine mountain streams tasted. He now is in your office complaining of a change in bowel habits. He reports 3–4 loose, foul-smelling stools each day with increased flatus and generalized abdominal discomfort.

Which of the following is the <u>most</u> appropriate next step in patient care?

    A. Counsel him that the symptoms are likely related to excess food and wine consumed during the trip, and he should spontaneously improve.
    B. Send stool for fecal leukocytes.
    C. Send a CBC to evaluate for eosinophilia.
    D. Send a *Giardia* specific antigen on the stool and begin empiric metronidazole.

37.

A family is enjoying a cruise of the lower Caribbean islands. All members of the family went on a shore excursion and visited a local restaurant. They all ate off the "exotic Caribbean" buffet. Four of five members of the family became ill almost simultaneously about 2 hours after eating. All developed nausea with profuse vomiting. All ill family members ate salad greens, rice, and cold macaroni salad. No one else on the cruise ship is currently experiencing these symptoms.

Which of the following is the <u>most</u> likely pathogen?

A. Norovirus (formerly known as Norwalk virus) gastroenteritis
B. Enterohemorrhagic *E. coli*
C. *Vibrio vulnificus*
D. *Bacillus cereus*

38.

You are asked to see a 23-year-old female patient on the psychiatric ward who has ingested a foreign body. Scout film demonstrates the item in the patient's esophagus.

Which of the following places her at greatest risk?

A. A fork
B. A lithium battery
C. A chicken bone
D. A paper clip
E. A copper coin

39.

A 39-year-old female with a persistent history of abdominal pain is evaluated for right upper quadrant tenderness. She has no history of alcohol consumption or tobacco/drug abuse, takes no medications, and has no history of previous hepatitis. She took oral contraceptives for a short while in her mid-20s but developed headaches and discontinued them. During the evaluation, an abdominal contrast tomography reports fatty infiltrates in the liver.

Past medical history: 2 normal pregnancies and deliveries at ages 26 and 28
Family history: Maternal hypertension
She currently has an implanted IUD for contraception.

Physical exam: Normal BMI = 33 (obese)

Laboratory results: Normals:
AST: 75   0–35 U/L
ALT: 90   0–35 U/L
Alk phos: 90   36–92 U/L
Albumin: 3.9   3.5–5.5 g/dL
INR: 1.0
BMP: normal
Urinalysis: normal
HbA1c: 4.0 %

Which of the following is the <u>most</u> appropriate next step in patient care?

    A. Removal of the IUD.
    B. Recommend she begin a weight-loss program.
    C. Perform a liver biopsy.
    D. Order HLA-B27.
    E. Reassure and offer continued follow-up.

40.

A 35-year-old male IV drug abuser presents with new onset of jaundice. His immunization history is unknown.

Laboratory returns with the following results:
Anti-HAV IgM: Negative
Anti-HAV IgG: Positive
HBcAb-IgM: Negative
HBcAb-IgG: Positive
HBsAg: Positive
Anti-HDV IgM: Positive
Anti-HDV IgG: Negative

Which of the following is the <u>most</u> likely diagnosis?

    A. Acute hepatitis A infection.
    B. He has never had a hepatitis A infection.
    C. Hepatitis D infection.
    D. He has recovered from a recent hepatitis D infection.
    E. Acute hepatitis A, acute hepatitis B, and acute hepatitis D infection.

41.

A 45-year-old male is accompanied to the clinic by his wife. He complains of difficulty swallowing for several years, but his wife has become increasingly concerned about his choking, particularly when eating with guests in a restaurant. It is non-painful and intermittent but occurs most frequently when he is eating meat. Other solids are usually but not always tolerated. He has never had difficulty with liquids. He denies any reflux or heartburn symptoms. He has had no weight loss.

Which of the following is the <u>most</u> likely diagnosis?

    A. Achalasia
    B. Schatzki ring
    C. Diffuse esophageal spasm
    D. Barrett esophagus
    E. Celiac sprue

42.

A 30-year-old woman presents with multiple complaints including fatigue, arthralgia, and a skin rash. She has seen several physicians and has been diagnosed only with dermatitis herpetiformis. She reports intermittent watery stools of increased frequency (sometimes > 12 stools/24 hours). She often has to flush the toilet several times due to the bulk of her bowel movements. On occasion, she experiences anorexia and abdominal distension. She has normal menstrual cycles but describes them as "heavy."

Physical exam is normal today. She has an iron deficiency anemia on laboratory testing.

Which of the following is the <u>most</u> likely diagnosis?

    A. Fibromyalgia
    B. Crohn disease
    C. Irritable bowel syndrome
    D. Celiac disease
    E. Dermatitis herpetiformis with psychosomatic components

43.

You evaluate a 17-year-old boy who has been generally healthy all of his life. He has a history of acne and was prescribed doxycycline. He presents now with a sudden onset of pain with swallowing of both liquids and solids that has been present for 2 days. He is weak and having difficulty sleeping because of the discomfort. He has not suffered heartburn in the past. His physical exam is significant for the moderate distress and bloodshot eyes from lack of sleep.

Which of the following is the <u>most</u> appropriate next step?

    A. EGD
    B. Trial of proton pump inhibitor
    C. Hyoscyamine PO before meals
    D. Upper GI, x-ray, and HIV assay
    E. Supportive care

44.

A 30-year-old woman presents with abdominal pain that is relieved by defecation. Her stools alternate from hard to loose and watery, and she frequently has to strain with incomplete evacuation. She reports abdominal distention occurring at least 3 times a week. Nocturnal symptoms occur frequently.

Which of her symptoms suggests a diagnosis other than irritable bowel syndrome?

    A. Abdominal pain relieved by defecation
    B. Stools alternate from hard to loose and watery
    C. Increased incidence of straining with incomplete evacuation
    D. Abdominal distention
    E. Frequent nocturnal symptoms

45.

A 37-year-old man presents for evaluation. He has been in good health all his life until 1 year ago. At that time, he noted he would have nocturnal episodes of wheezing. Gradually, these episodes became worse, and he was prescribed beta-agonists. Recently another physician added long-acting inhaled steroids. He reports no improvement in his symptoms.

He describes episodes of awakening several hours after going to sleep with cough and prolonged wheezing. He has no previous history of asthma and no known allergies.

Today, on physical examination, you do not hear any wheezing.

Which of the following diagnostic studies would be __most__ appropriate?

    A. Upper endoscopy
    B. Peak flow measurement
    C. Lung CT scan
    D. 24-hour ambulatory esophageal pH probe
    E. Barium swallow

PULMONARY MEDICINE

46.

A 25-year-old female presents to your office for initial evaluation of her asthma. She reports she was diagnosed with asthma 3 years ago. Her symptoms include daily cough that is nonproductive and seems to be worse at night. She has occasional wheezing and some dyspnea on exertion when exercising. She has been prescribed a short-acting beta-agonist that she uses 4–5 times daily with relief that lasts about 30–60 minutes.

She has no other significant past medical history. Her sister also has asthma. She denies any smoking history. She has 2 dogs at home and has never had allergy testing. She has no symptoms of reflux.

Which of the following is the next best step in management for this patient?

A. Start once-daily oral leukotriene receptor antagonist.
B. Start a low-dose inhaled corticosteroid.
C. Start a long-acting beta-agonist.
D. Start a proton pump inhibitor every night.
E. Continue current treatment regimen with short-acting beta-agonist.

47.

A 65-year-old male presents to the emergency department with acute shortness of breath. He complains of pain in his right chest that is worse with deep inspiration. He also reports some lightheadedness but no syncope. These symptoms started to occur 2 hours prior to presentation and awoke him from sleep. He does report that he recently returned from an overseas airplane trip that lasted 6 hours. He denies any lower extremity edema.

On exam: P: 125, BP: 130/45, T: 37.1° C, RR: 24   Oxygen sats: 88% on room air

He is in mild distress without accessory muscle use. His lungs are clear to auscultation. Cardiac exam reveals tachycardia with regular rhythm, no murmurs. The remainder of his exam is unremarkable. ECG reveals sinus tachycardia with right bundle-branch block.

A CXR is read as: "No significant cardiopulmonary process."

Which of the following should be done next?

A. Start low-dose aspirin orally.
B. Obtain chest CT angiogram.
C. Start PO warfarin at 10 mg daily.
D. Start empiric antibiotics for pneumonia.
E. Discharge home with NSAIDs with follow-up with primary care physician in 1 week.

48.

A 54-year-old man is brought to your office by his wife. She complains that he snores loudly every night, and this keeps her awake. She also notices that her husband sleeps restlessly and sometimes seems to suddenly awaken himself from sleep. He complains of morning headaches and a dry mouth every morning. He currently weighs 229 lbs, which is about a 32-lb weight gain since his last visit one year ago. His current BMI is 34.

He has no other significant past medical history. His blood pressure is 140/90.

Which of the following is <u>false</u> about obstructive sleep apnea (OSA)?

    A. Neck circumference > 16 cm increases the risk of obstructive sleep apnea.
    B. Treatment of OSA can reverse hypertension without any additional medications.
    C. An apnea-hypopnea index (AHI) greater than 1 (one) is consistent with a diagnosis of OSA.
    D. CPAP (continuous positive airway pressure) is the most commonly used treatment for OSA.
    E. Untreated OSA increases the risk for coronary artery disease.

49.

A 35-year-old female presents to the emergency department with complaints of shortness of breath for 3 days. She has had a dry cough, fever, and chills. Her symptoms of shortness of breath have progressed very rapidly such that she cannot walk from room to room without difficulty. She has no significant past medical history and works as a waitress in a diner. She is a nonsmoker and denies any illicit drug use.

On presentation, she is in marked respiratory distress.
P: 125, BP: 90/45, Oxygen sats: 79% Room air, T: 39.4° C, RR: 38
She has marked accessory muscle use. Lung exam reveals diffuse bilateral crackles and coarse rhonchi. She has a tachycardic rhythm and no peripheral edema.
CXR reveals bilateral alveolar infiltrates without cardiomegaly or pleural effusions. Echocardiogram reveals normal LVEF, mild TR, and moderate elevation of pulmonary artery systolic pressures.
Her WBC is elevated to 18,000. Her renal function is normal. Blood cultures are now growing *Streptococcus pneumoniae*.

The patient is intubated and placed on mechanical ventilation. Her initial ABG on 100% F_iO_2 is: pH: 7.29, pCO_2: 58, pO_2: 74, HCO_3: 21.

Which of the following is associated with a reduction in mortality in this condition?

    A. Initiation of high-dose corticosteroids
    B. Use of neuromuscular blockade during ventilation
    C. Mechanical ventilation with tidal volumes set at 6–8 mL/kg of ideal body weight
    D. Placement of the patient in the prone position.
    E. Use of nitric oxide during ventilation

50.

A 72-year-old male comes in for follow-up evaluation. He has a known history of emphysema. He complains of persistent shortness of breath with exertion, which he says is getting worse. He can only walk about half a block on flat ground prior to getting dyspneic. He is significantly impaired with steps. He smoked 1 pack per day for 45 years and still smokes about 1/2 pack per day. He denies any exertional chest pain, palpitations, or lower extremity edema. His current medications include tiotropium bromide q day, salmeterol/fluticasone combination discus bid, and albuterol MDI qid.

On exam: P: 100 RR: 28 Oxygen saturations on RA: 89%   110/65
Wt.: 52 kg (decreased by 3 kg since last visit)
Lungs: severely diminished breath sounds bilaterally, prolonged exhalation, no wheezing
His PFTs are as follows:

FVC: 2.05 L (65% predicted)
FEV_1: .087   (35% predicted)
FEV_1/FVC: 55%
TLC: 4.12 L (125% predicted)
DLCO: 11.2 (45% predicted)

Which of the following should be offered to this patient next?

    A. Oxygen determination with rest, exercise, and nocturnally.
    B. Influenza vaccine annually.
    C. Referral to pulmonary rehabilitation.
    D. Smoking cessation program.
    E. All of the choices are correct.

51.

You are asked to evaluate a patient due to their shortness of breath. He is 74 years old with a history of coronary artery disease with CABG eight years prior. He reports exertional dyspnea, difficulty breathing when lying flat, and increased lower extremity edema. A chest radiograph is done and reveals a moderately sized, right-sided pleural effusion. On your examination, he had diminished breath sounds along the lower right portion of the right lung with dullness to percussion along the lower right back. A thoracentesis is performed and 900 mL of clear, straw-colored fluid is removed.

Pleural Fluid:	Serum:	
Protein: 1.9	Protein: 4.2	
LDH: 120	LDH: 315	
pH: 7.30	WBC: 200; RBC: 0	
Gram stain: no organisms		

[handwritten: 4.2 / 1.9 = 2 ; 315 / 120 = 2.7 = Exud.]

Two days later a CXR is repeated, and the effusion is still present, although slightly smaller. The patient is comfortable and not in any distress.

What should be done next?

    A. Repeat thoracentesis
    B. Placement of a large bore chest tube
    C. Placement of a small bore chest tube
    D. Cardiac catheterization
    E. Echocardiogram

52.

A 24-year-old male who lives in southwestern Ohio comes to the emergency department complaining of a rash on his legs. He reports that these "red bumps" erupted about 1 week ago, and they are becoming more painful. He has no significant past medical history and is a nonsmoker. He has no recent exposures to any new dusts, chemicals, detergents, etc. He also denies any new medications. He did eat shrimp about 10 days ago but does this often and has never had any reactions. He has never been allergy tested, but he has never had any food-related reactions.

His rash appears below:

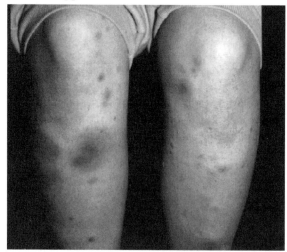

On a previous emergency department visit, he had a chest radiograph done for cough about 2 months prior, which is also below.

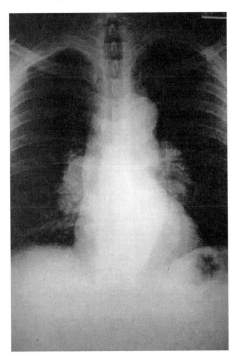

What is the <u>most</u> likely diagnosis?

A. Poison ivy
B. Histoplasmosis
C. Allergic reaction to shellfish
D. Berylliosis
E. Sarcoidosis

53.

A 43-year-old female is referred to your office for an abnormal chest CT. About 3 weeks ago, she had RUQ abdominal pain and underwent an abdominal CT. She was diagnosed with cholecystitis and underwent a laparoscopic cholecystectomy. An incidental finding of an oval-shaped right lower lobe lung nodule was noted. It is characterized as calcified and about 3 x 4 mm in size. A chest CT was then performed that confirmed these findings without any other abnormalities.

The patient has a PMH notable for hypertension for which she takes an ACE inhibitor. She is a lifelong nonsmoker and works in an office environment. There is no family history of malignancy.

What would you recommend for this patient?

A. Referral to a thoracic surgeon for surgical resection of the nodule.
B. CT guided biopsy of nodule.
C. Obtain a PET scan.
D. Repeat chest CT scan every 6 months for a total of 2 years to ensure stability.
E. Reassurance with no further follow-up

54.

An 81-year-old female has severe emphysema with severe dyspnea on exertion. She is on 4 L oxygen continuously. She has difficulty with performing her activities of daily living (ADLs). She uses an inhaled long-acting anti-cholinergic, an inhaled long-acting beta-agonist/inhaled steroid combination, and oral theophylline. She has been to pulmonary rehabilitation. She asks your opinion about surgical options for her COPD.

Which of the following is true?

A. Lung volume reduction surgery has been shown to increase mortality in all patients who undergo the procedure.

B. Lung volume reduction surgery has been shown to decrease mortality in all patients who undergo the procedure.

C. Lung volume reduction surgery improves outcomes in patients with predominantly upper-lobe disease and very low exercise capacity.

D. This patient should be considered for lung transplantation.

55.

A 62-year-old male presents with a 3-year history of dyspnea on exertion. He has a chronic dry cough without any specific triggers. He is a lifelong nonsmoker and spent most of his working life in a chemical plant dealing with petroleum. His oxygen saturation at rest is 93% but decreases to 86% with exertion after 3 minutes. He has digital clubbing but no cyanosis or edema. His lung exam reveals dry, coarse inspiratory crackles without wheezing. A chest CT is performed. It reveals bibasilar fibrosis with traction bronchiectasis and subpleural blebs without any ground glass abnormalities. The patient is sent for surgical lung biopsy, and the pathology is read as "UIP pattern with fibroblastic foci, temporal heterogeneity, honeycombing appearance, and minimal inflammation."

What is the most likely diagnosis?

A. Sarcoidosis
B. Acute respiratory distress syndrome
C. Emphysema
D. Idiopathic pulmonary fibrosis
E. Asbestosis

56.

A 16-year-old male presents to your office with complaints of wheezing on exertion. He has recently started cross-country track and notes wheezing at the height of his exercise that often remains for several hours after activity. He has tried his friend's asthma inhaler but can't tell if it helps. He denies smoking.

PMH: Good health except for prolonged ICU stay for Guillain-Barré syndrome at age 12.
Normal physical exam.

Which of the following is the <u>most</u> appropriate course of action?

A. Prescribe a short-acting beta-agonist before starting exercise.
B. Prescribe cromolyn sodium as prophylaxis for exercise-induced asthma.
C. Perform PFTs with a flow-volume loop.
D. Perform fluoroscopy of the diaphragm to document residual paralysis.

57.

A 26-year-old female with asthma presents to your office for routine follow-up. She was diagnosed with asthma at age 16 and required ICU admission once at age 17. She has never been on a ventilator. She is adherent to her asthma regimen. Review of systems is positive for daily wheezing, requiring inhaled bronchodilators, and nocturnal coughing 3x/week that wake her from sleep.

Meds:
Beclomethasone 80 mcg bid
Albuterol MDI prn

PE:
Normal vital signs
No jugular venous distention
Lungs with symmetric expansion, resonant to percussion, clear to auscultation

Which of the following is the <u>most</u> appropriate next step in patient care?

A. Add ipratropium bromide bid.
B. Add salmeterol bid.
C. Increase beclomethasone to 320 mcg bid.
D. Add theophylline.
E. Add montelukast daily.

58.

A 36-year-old woman has had increasing dyspnea for 8 years. She has no cough or increased sputum production. On physical exam, there is hyperresonance to percussion in the bases. A chest radiograph reveals increased lung volumes with flattening of the diaphragmatic leaves bilaterally.

Which of the following laboratory findings is she <u>most</u> likely to have?

A. Positive methacholine challenge test
B. Increased sweat chloride
C. Decreased alpha-1-antitrypsin
D. Elevated serum iron stores
E. Decreased ceruloplasmin

59.

A 32-year-old female presents to your office complaining of wheezing for 2 weeks. At her last appointment 6 weeks ago, she was noted to have intentionally lost weight through an exercise program, and she requested to be taken off two of her medications, cimetidine and acyclovir. She was in a good state of health until developing cold symptoms two weeks ago, and since then, she has wheezed daily. She denies tobacco, drugs, or alcohol. She has not had any fever. The cold symptoms have since resolved.

PMH:
Asthma since childhood, previously stable x 5 years on her current regimen
GERD
Genital herpes

Meds: theophylline, cimetidine (discontinued), acyclovir (discontinued), beclomethasone high-dose bid, salmeterol bid, montelukast qd, albuterol PRN

At her last appointment, her theophylline level was 17 mg/dL (therapeutic range: 10–20 mg/dL)

Which of the following is the <u>most</u> likely cause of her persistent wheezing?

    A. Underlying interstitial lung disease
    B. Decreased serum theophylline concentration
    C. Undiagnosed *Bordetella pertussis*
    D. Antagonistic drug interaction between theophylline and montelukast
    E. Tachyphylaxis to salmeterol

60.

A 65-year-old male insulation worker has a chest radiograph that shows bilateral pleural plaques along the lateral chest walls. He was exposed to asbestos intermittently during his occupational pursuits. He is asymptomatic, and his physical exam is unremarkable. He does not smoke.

What is the <u>most</u> appropriate next step in patient care?

    A. Pulmonary function tests to determine if plaques are causing restriction
    B. CT scan of the chest to determine if plaques contain calcium
    C. Bronchoscopy with biopsy to check for pulmonary fibrosis
    D. Tuberculin skin test with standard strength PPD
    E. Observation and reassurance

61.

A 42-year-old man presents to your office complaining of cough, wheezing, and shortness of breath that has been progressive for the past 3 months. PMH is negative, and he takes no medications. He works in private practice as an attorney and has been in a monogamous marriage for 17 years. He drinks 1 glass of wine nightly and denies the use of tobacco or drugs.

PE: Normal vital signs
Normal exam except for diffuse fine crackles auscultated in the lung bases

CXR: Diffuse interstitial infiltrates

Which of the following is the <u>most</u> appropriate next step in patient care?

    A. Prescribe albuterol by MDI.
    B. Begin prednisone 60 mg daily.
    C. Order a sweat test.
    D. Schedule a high-resolution CT scan of the chest.
    E. Refer to the pulmonologist for bronchoscopy.

62.

A 29-year-old woman has an x-ray film of the chest that shows bilateral prominent pulmonary arteries without pulmonary congestion. She has fatigue and chest discomfort with exertion. Physical examination shows a large *a* wave in the jugular pulse, clear lung fields, a systolic lift along the left sternal border, and a split S_2 audible at the left sternal border and apex, with a loud second component. No cardiac murmur is present.

Which of the following tests is <u>most</u> likely to provide the correct diagnosis?

    A. Pulmonary function with flow-volume loops
    B. Echocardiogram
    C. CT angiogram with PE protocol
    D. High-resolution CT of the chest
    E. Bronchoscopy with bronchoalveolar lavage

63.

A 28-year-old male smoker presents to the emergency department with complaints of a swollen and painful left leg. He states he was in good health until 1 week ago when he began to notice a dull pain in his leg. Since then, he has experienced swelling and redness. He denies trauma to the leg.

Doppler ultrasound reveals a left popliteal thrombosis.

Which of the following is the <u>most</u> likely cause of his DVT?

    A. Protein S deficiency
    B. Homocysteinemia
    C. Occult malignancy
    D. Antithrombin III deficiency
    E. *Factor V Leiden* gene mutation (activated protein C resistance)

64.

A 58-year-old woman has had pain and tenderness of the long bones of the lower extremities, knees, and ankles for 2 months. She has smoked one pack of cigarettes daily for 30 years. She has had rheumatoid arthritis for 15 years. Examination of the lower extremities shows tenderness to palpation of the femur and tibia bilaterally and slight warmth and tenderness of the knees and ankles. X-ray films show periosteal new bone formation of the femurs.

Her symptoms are <u>most</u> likely a complication of which of the following?

A. Rheumatoid arthritis
B. Squamous cell carcinoma
C. Small cell lung cancer
D. Osteoporosis
E. Adenocarcinoma of the lung

65.

A 45-year-old man with interstitial pulmonary fibrosis (IPF) returns to your office for routine follow-up after receiving his diagnosis 2 months prior. He continues on prednisone and cyclophosphamide and says, "I feel great!" He states he is certain he will be one of the few who does well with this diagnosis because he has had a "dramatic response."

Physical exam is unchanged.

Repeat HRCT shows persistent ground-glass opacities.

Which of the following is associated with physiologic improvement of IPF after treatment?

A. Development of diabetes secondary to steroid use
B. Improvement of the ground glass on HRCT
C. Improvement in lung pathology
D. Subjective improvement in dyspnea
E. Reduction of the A-a gradient with exercise

66.

A 60-year-old man has had a cough with production of sputum for the past month. He is afebrile with decreased breath sounds at the right lung base. A chest radiograph reveals an area of consolidation in the right lower lobe with air bronchograms. He is given antibiotic therapy; but when he is seen 2 months later, the chest radiograph is unchanged, and his cough continues. Sputum is clear but has a "salty" taste.

Which of the following is the <u>most</u> likely diagnosis?

A. Unresolved *Mycoplasma pneumoniae*
B. Tuberculosis
C. Lipoid pneumonia from aspiration
D. Bronchoalveolar cell carcinoma
E. Obstructive pneumonia from squamous cell carcinoma

67.

A usually healthy 38-year-old woman comes to the physician because of a 3-day history of pain and swelling of her right leg. She has smoked one pack of cigarettes daily for 20 years. Her only medication is oral contraceptives. Her pulse is 78/min and regular. Her right calf is edematous and tender. The peripheral arterial pulses are present and normal in upstroke. Venous duplex ultrasonography shows that the superficial and deep femoral veins are not compressible.

Which of the following is the most appropriate next step in management?

A. Thrombolytic therapy
B. Observation
C. Low-molecular-weight heparin therapy
D. Insertion of a vena cava filter
E. V/Q scan

68.

A 24-year-old African-American male applies for work in the steel mill. He has a negative health history and a normal ROS. A routine CXR is performed and sent for your review.

Which of the following is the most appropriate next step in patient care?

A. Order a contrasted CT of the chest, abdomen, and pelvis.
B. Collect 3 sputum samples for acid-fast smears and cultures, and send one sample for *M. tuberculosis* nucleic acid amplification.
C. Order high-resolution CT scan of the chest.
D. Start prednisone 60 mg qd.
E. Start work on Monday.

69.

A 62-year-old male presents to your office for follow-up. He has a history of COPD but has had no recent testing. He complains of chronic dyspnea on exertion walking on flat ground after 50 feet as well as shortness of breath with stairs. He has not previously been intubated and was hospitalized twice in the last six months for respiratory issues. His only respiratory-related medication included albuterol q6h as needed for dyspnea. He is an active smoker with a 50-pack-year history of smoking.

Pulmonary Function Tests were performed:
FEV_1: 1.5L (49% predicted)
FVC: 3.0L (64% predicted)
FEV_1/FVC: 50%
Oximetry Testing: Resting, Room Air: > 95%
Exercise, Room Air: > 93%
Overnight, Room Air: > 91%

Based on current evidence, which of the following would <u>not</u> be beneficial for this patient?

    A. Smoking cessation
    B. Use of oxygen at 2 LPM daily with rest and exertion
    C. Pulmonary rehabilitation
    D. Daily use of an inhaled corticosteroid
    E. Annual influenza vaccine

70.

A 52-year-old female initially complained of cough and fever. She was seen in the emergency department and was noted to have significant respiratory distress. Her O_2 sats were 84% on 100% non-rebreather mask. Due to continued respiratory distress, the patient was intubated and placed on mechanical ventilation. Her initial ABG post-intubation is:

pH: 7.28 P_aO_2: 59 P_aCO_2: 54 O_2 Sats: 89% F_iO_2: 100%
Mechanical Ventilator settings: AC mode, Rate 20, F_iO_2: 100%   Tidal volume: 550, PEEP 8
Vitals: T: 39.1° C P: 120 BP: 100/44 RR: 24
Her CXR reveals diffuse bilateral infiltrates.
Echocardiogram reveals an estimated LVEF of 55% without any significant valvular abnormalities.

Which of the following has been shown to improve mortality in those with this condition?

    A. Placement of a right heart catheter to assess cardiac parameters
    B. Use of nitric oxide
    C. Maintenance of tidal volumes at 6 mL/kg of ideal body weight
    D. Maintenance of tidal volumes at 12 mL/kg/hour
    E. Initiation of systemic corticosteroids after 5 days of ventilatory support

71.

A 54-year-old male who resides in Ohio presents with a 6-month history of recurrent cough that is nonproductive. He reports that the cough is persistent and worse during the day and seems to improve during the night. It has been persistent, but it seemed to improve when he took a vacation to Florida two months ago and recurred on his return. He denies any sputum, wheezing, reflux symptoms, chest pain, edema, orthopnea, paroxysmal nocturnal dyspnea, or palpitations. He does endorse mild dyspnea on exertion, as well as occasional fevers without chills. He has no recent sick contacts or travel exposure. He denies any smoking or illicit drug use. He began working for a mushroom farm 9 months ago. Prior to that, he worked on various construction jobs and was told that there was some asbestos material exposure, but he is not sure how much. Chest radiograph is ordered and reveals patchy infiltrates in the right upper lobe and left lingula region, without any effusions or masses.

Which of the following is the next best step in management for this patient?

    A. Bronchoscopy with transbronchial biopsy
    B. Initiation of corticosteroids at 1 mg/kg daily
    C. Transthoracic echocardiogram
    D. Prolonged duration away from his work environment
    E. Start empiric treatment with oral fluoroquinolone.

72.

A 29-year-old female is 32-weeks pregnant with her first gestation. She presents to the emergency department with a 2-day history of acute shortness of breath and left-sided chest pain. She describes the pain as sharp, located in the mid axilla along the 6th to 8th rib location. She denies any recent trauma. She further denies any fevers, chills, syncope, cough, or sputum production. Her legs are swollen and have been progressively increasing in size over the last 4 weeks of her pregnancy, but they are equal in size and without erythema.

Upon presentation her vitals: T: 99.1° F, P: 125
RR: 24 BP: 100/45 O_2 Sats: 92% on room air.
She is without any respiratory distress. Her exam is notable for a regular tachycardia and a gravid uterus appropriate for stage of gestation. Lungs are clear to auscultation. She has 1+ lower extremity edema without any asymmetry.
There is no sign of fetal distress.
Chest radiograph is without any abnormalities, and EKG reveals a sinus tachycardia.
Lower extremity venous Doppler ultrasound reveals an acute deep venous thrombosis in the left common femoral vein.

Which of the following is the next best step in treatment?

    A. Obtain a ventilation-perfusion scan.
    B. Begin unfractionated heparin by continuous infusion according to weight.
    C. Initiate therapy with low molecular weight heparin at 1 mg/kg SQ q12 with concomitant warfarin therapy.
    D. Initiate aspirin therapy.
    E. Stat C-section for emergent delivery.

73.

A 72-year-old male with a history of coronary artery disease and systolic cardiomyopathy presents with a 2-week history of progressive shortness of breath associated with a dry cough. He also complains of 2+ lower extremity edema. On lung exam, there are decreased breath sounds throughout the lower 2/3 of his right lung with dullness to percussion. Chest x-ray reveals a moderate pleural effusion. The patient undergoes bedside thoracentesis with the removal of 800 mL of clear, straw-colored fluid. Studies sent:

Pleural fluid: Protein 1.3 LDH: 130
Culture: No growth
Serum: Protein 4.2   LDH: 290

This improves the patient's symptoms, but a repeat chest x-ray four days later reveals recurrent pleural fluid.

What should be done next for this patient?

    A. Placement of large bore chest tube for continued drainage
    B. More aggressive treatment for congestive heart failure with diuretics
    C. Thoracic surgery consult for pleurodesis
    D. Repeat thoracentesis

74.

A 67-year-old male presents with complaints of shortness of breath. It has been occurring for years, but he has noticed it more over the last six months. He complains of exertional dyspnea not associated with any chest pain but does have some occasional dry cough. He smokes 1 pack per day and has been doing so since age 31. His only other significant past medical history includes hypertension and diabetes. His examination reveals a normal cardiac exam with distant breath sounds on lung auscultation without any adventitial sounds. Chest radiograph reveals mild hyperexpansion and mild cardiomegaly without any other major abnormalities. He is sent for pulmonary function tests:

	Actual	Predicted
FVC	2.2 L	51%
FEV_1	0.98 L	31%
FEV_1/FVC	44%	
TLC	7.51 L	125%
DLCO	9.03 mL/min/mmHg	25%

The pattern seen on pulmonary function testing is _most_ consistent with which of the following?

- A. Very severe obstructive airways disease with hyperinflation
- B. Moderate obstructive airways disease without hyperinflation
- C. Moderate restrictive disease
- D. Isolated reduction in diffusion capacity related to pulmonary vascular disease
- E. Mixed restrictive and obstructive pattern

75.

A 72-year-old male who is a nursing home resident is brought to the emergency department due to fever to 39.1° C. Upon presentation, he is noted to have a heart rate of 125 and a blood pressure of 75/42. Urinalysis reveals many WBCs, and many bacteria and cultures are drawn.

He appears to be in moderate distress and has moderate diffuse abdominal pain. He is fairly lethargic and barely arouses to verbal or painful stimuli. Initial labs drawn reveal a lactate level of 4.2, WBC of 23.5, and Hgb of 10.4.

Which of the following would not be indicated in the treatment of this patient?

- A. Early initiation of empiric antibiotics
- B. Delivery of crystalloid fluid to target a central venous pressure of 8–12 mmHg
- C. Placement of a central venous catheter
- D. Initiation of drotrecogin alfa (activated) by continuous IV infusion for 96 hours
- E. Admission to the intensive care unit

76.

A 23-year-old female has a history of asthma since age 16. She reports symptoms of dry cough and exertional dyspnea. Her cough is worse at night but also worsens with cold air. She has symptoms almost every night. She has an inhaler of albuterol that she uses nightly and as needed for increased shortness of breath. She denies smoking, has no pets, and currently is a full-time student. She has not noticed any seasonal variation or any worsening with different environments. She denies symptoms of reflux.

What is the next best step in management?

A. Start treatment with a medium dose inhaled corticosteroid along with albuterol as needed.
B. Start treatment with a long-acting beta-agonist along with albuterol as needed.
C. Refer for allergy testing.
D. Initiate treatment with a proton pump inhibitor nightly.

77.

A 54-year-old male with moderate COPD presents to the emergency department with a 4-day history of progressive shortness of breath. He is noted to be lethargic and in respiratory distress with accessory muscle use and a respiratory rate of 36. He has poor air movement without any wheezing.

The patient is intubated and placed on mechanical ventilator support with the following settings:
Mode: Assist control ventilator rate (set): 14
Patient spontaneous rate: 22
Tidal volume: 450 mL F_iO_2: 100%
PEEP: 5 cm
An arterial blood gas is obtained:
pH: 7.22 pCO_2: 64 P_aO_2: 240 HCO_3: 22

Which of the following would help improve the pH?

A. Increase the set rate on the ventilator to 22 breaths per minute.
B. Start continuous infusion of bicarbonate mixed in dextrose 5%.
C. Decrease the F_iO_2 to 50%.
D. Deeper sedation to decrease respiratory rate to 14.
E. Increase the tidal volume 500 mL.

78.

A 33-year-old woman in your clinic has a chest CT (see below). She has mild, worsening airflow limitation on serial spirometry. She has increasing exertional dyspnea that is now significantly limiting her activity. She had a small, spontaneous pneumothorax last year that resolved without intervention. She has never smoked, but her spouse does smoke.

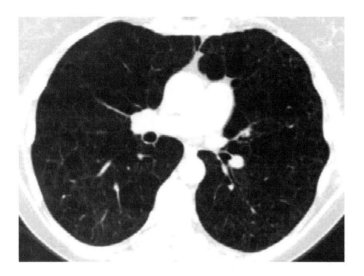

The <u>most</u> likely diagnosis is which of the following?

    A. Advanced emphysema from secondhand smoke
    B. Alpha-1-antitrypsin deficiency with advanced emphysema
    C. Lymphangioleiomyomatosis (LAM)
    D. Asthma
    E. Idiopathic pulmonary fibrosis

79.

A 67-year-old man with Type 2 diabetes mellitus, obesity, and hypertension is admitted for elective colonoscopy for chronic iron deficient anemia. He undergoes a prepped colonoscopy and receives midazolam 1 mg and fentanyl 25 µg. His eyelids close, and he does not respond to voice. Within a few minutes, the nurse reports that the patient's pulse oximetry reading is falling. He is making an effort to breathe, but there are paradoxical movements of the chest and abdomen. Vital signs, including temperature and blood pressure, remain stable. The patient is suctioned, but scant material is recovered. Chest radiograph does not reveal acute infiltrates.

What is the <u>most</u> likely cause of this patient's response to conscious sedation?

    A. Aspiration pneumonitis
    B. Hemorrhagic shock
    C. Obstructive sleep apnea (OSA)
    D. Sepsis
    E. Decreased respiratory drive due to sedation

80.

A 29-year-old woman is admitted to the hospital with a 1-week history of nonproductive cough, shortness of breath, and dyspnea on exertion. She is only able to walk a room's length before she needs to rest. Further symptoms include fever and chills. She has a known history of HIV disease and previous CD4+ cell count was 10 cells/µL ten months ago. She has otherwise been noncompliant with follow-up visits and has not been on any treatment for her HIV disease.

On examination, the patient is in mild respiratory distress. Vital signs: T: 39.2° C, BP: 121/62
HR: 127 RR: 25
Pulse ox saturation: 88% on room air. She has a white exudate throughout the posterior oropharynx as well as on her tongue. Cardiovascular examination reveals tachycardia with regular rate and rhythm and no murmurs. Lung examination reveals diffuse crackles with poor air movement throughout.

Labs reveal a normal WBC count and basic metabolic panel. Lactate dehydrogenase (LDH) is elevated by three times the normal range. Her P_aO_2 is 60. Chest x-ray is below. Bronchoscopy with BAL is performed, and the results are pending.

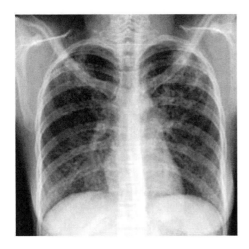

What is the best step in management for this patient?

A. Amphotericin B
B. Isoniazid, ethambutol, rifampin, and pyrazinamide
C. Trimethoprim/sulfamethoxazole (TMP/SMX)
D. TMP/SMX and prednisone
E. Vancomycin

81.

A 57-year-old man with a history of obesity and hypertension presents to the emergency department complaining of dizziness, weakness, and dyspnea on exertion. This has been occurring for one day but continues to escalate. He denies chest pain or calf tenderness. He recently traveled overseas on a 6-hour flight and returned seven days prior to presentation.

Physical examination reveals: HR: 105, BP: 132/76, RR: 22, 87% oxygen saturations on room air.
Chest radiograph is unremarkable, and the EKG reveals sinus tachycardia. Chest CT angiogram demonstrates a saddle pulmonary embolus in the main pulmonary arterial trunk. Transthoracic echocardiogram reveals evidence of acute right heart strain, with moderate reduction in the right ventricular systolic function. There is also tricuspid regurgitation with pulmonary hypertension. Computed tomography of the head is normal and reveals no cause for dizziness. He has no known contraindications to anticoagulation.

How should the echocardiographic findings of right ventricular strain alter management of this patient?

A. The patient is at increased risk for shock or death from PE and should receive more intensive monitoring.
B. The patient is at increased risk for shock or death from PE and should receive thrombolytic therapy.
C. The patient is at increased risk for recurrent PE and should receive LMWH rather than warfarin.
D. The patient is at increased risk for ongoing embolization and should receive a vena caval interruption device.

82.

A 65-year-old man presents to his physician's office with a 6-month history of wheezing, dyspnea on exertion, and daily sputum production. He is a 50-pack-year smoker but is otherwise healthy. Examination shows markedly decreased breath sounds with mild wheezing at the end of expiration.

Spirometry is performed:
FVC is 2.3 L.
FEV_1 is 1.5 L (60% of predicted).
The FEV_1/FVC ratio is 65%.

Which of the following interventions will be **most** effective for improving this patient's long-term survival?

A. Inhaled corticosteroids
B. Long-term oral corticosteroids
C. Inhaled ipratropium
D. Smoking cessation

83.

An 18-year-old man comes to your office for follow-up examination. He has a known history of asthma since age 12. His PEF is 400 L/min (80% of personal best). He currently takes fluticasone 110 µg 2 puffs twice daily and uses an albuterol inhaler 3 to 4 times daily. He is compliant with his medications, but he still wakes up at night 3 to 4 times a week with coughing that is relieved with his albuterol inhaler.

Which of the following is the best management option for this patient?

A. Add a long-acting β-agonist such as salmeterol or formoterol to his fluticasone therapy.
B. Prescribe azithromycin 500 mg daily for seven days.
C. Prescribe prednisone 40 mg daily for 7 days.
D. Start therapy with omalizumab.
E. No change in treatment and reassurance.

84.

A 65-year-old male with poor general health status was evaluated in your office for progressive complaints of shortness of breath and decreasing exercise tolerance. As part of the workup, pulmonary function testing was ordered. The results of the testing revealed a significant decrease in the total lung capacity, functional reserve capacity, and the residual volume. The carbon monoxide diffusional capacity was found to be normal.

Which of the following diagnoses would be **most** consistent with these findings?

A. Silica pneumoconiosis
B. Ankylosing spondylitis
C. Procainamide-induced pneumonitis
D. Pulmonary sarcoidosis
E. Eosinophilic pneumonia

85.

Pulmonary ventilation, alveolar gas exchange, or combinations of these two elements can affect respiratory compromise.

Which of the following is **most** important in distinguishing between ventilatory failure and a gas exchange defect in a patient with breathing difficulties?

A. A-a gradient
B. P_aO_2 levels
C. Pulse oximetry
D. P_aCO_2
E. Serum pH

86.

Spirometry and peak flow measurement are two methods for evaluating airway status in pulmonary patients.

When considering the data available from these two modalities, the value obtained with a peak flow meter corresponds **most** directly to which spirometric equivalent?

A. Forced expiratory volume in 1 second (FEV_1)
B. Total lung capacity (TLC)
C. The first few milliseconds of airflow
D. Forced vital capacity (FVC)

87.

A 30-year-old male with history of asthma comes to the emergency department complaining that he "can't breathe."

He is diaphoretic, 140/90, HR 128, RR 30.

On physical exam the following is noted:
He has an "Inspiratory Fall in Blood Pressure."
He is leaning forward using his accessory muscles.
Hyperresonance and diffuse wheezes are found on chest exam.

ABG on room air: pH 7.39 pCO_2 45 mmHg pO_2 60 mmHg

Which of the following is the <u>most</u> appropriate next step in management?

    A. Magnesium sulfate IV
    B. Noninvasive mask ventilation
    C. 40% F_iO_2 by face mask
    D. Antibiotic therapy
    E. Intubation and mechanical ventilation

88.

A 52-year-old smoker presents for follow-up. He has stable dyspnea on exertion, but he notes new lower extremity edema.

PMH: CHD, HTN, COPD
PE: O_2 sat 89%
JVD, trace pedal edema
Barrel-shaped chest
Distant heart sounds, loud P_2
Left sternal holosystolic murmur
Wheezes

Which of the following is the <u>most</u> appropriate next step in patient care?

    A. Prescribe oxygen for use during ambulation.
    B. Order dobutamine stress test with nuclear images.
    C. Change metoprolol to an ACE inhibitor.
    D. Increase the beclomethasone dose.
    E. Prescribe oxygen for continuous use.

89.

A 25-year-old complains of "shortness of breath" that began at a social gathering. He complains of paresthesias of his hands and feet and developed left-sided pleuritic chest pain.

PMH: Major depression

On exam he is tachypneic.
ABG: pH 7.47, pCO_2 32, pO_2 92

Which of the following is the <u>most</u> likely diagnosis?

    A. Anaphylactoid reaction
    B. Hypersensitivity pneumonitis
    C. Asthma exacerbation
    D. Panic attack
    E. Pulmonary embolism

90.

A 56-year-old man is brought to the emergency department 2 hours after the onset of severe shortness of breath that began during a social gathering. He thinks perfume from a guest triggered his shortness of breath.

PMH: Major depressive disorder, hypertension, tobacco abuse (1½ ppd cigarettes x 30 years)

ROS: Stable early a.m. cough x 5 years and shortness of breath with exertion of 1 flight of stairs.

Meds: HCTZ 25 mg qd

PE: Moderate distress with RR 32, BP 138/86, afebrile

Normal PE except for tachypnea

ABG: pH 7.47, pCO$_2$ 32 mmHg, pO$_2$ 85 mmHg

CXR: Diffuse increase in lung markings, increased at the bases

Which of the following is the _most_ appropriate next step in patient care?

    A. Intramuscular injection of epinephrine for anaphylactoid reaction.
    B. Albuterol inhalation by metered-dose inhaler with a spacer.
    C. Albuterol and ipratropium inhalation by metered-dose inhaler with a spacer plus oral prednisone 60 mg.
    D. Helical CT scan.
    E. Change sertraline to paroxetine and recommend follow-up with his primary care provider in 72 hours.

91.

A 35-year-old woman presents complaining of dyspnea with exertion since delivering her baby 6 months earlier. She is a nonsmoker. Her recent pregnancy and delivery were uncomplicated. She owns a parakeet.

Her family history is significant for _Factor V Leiden_ gene mutation and venous thromboembolic events in several family members.

PE: Afebrile, BP 122/76, HR 82, RR 12, BMI 31
Well-nourished female in no respiratory distress
Distant breath sounds and trace edema in both feet and otherwise normal exam

ECG: Nonspecific T-wave changes, leads V4–V6
CXR: Normal
ABG: pH 7.45, pCO$_2$ 48, pO$_2$ 76
D-dimer: Normal range

Which of the following is the <u>most</u> likely diagnosis?

A. Primary pulmonary hypertension
B. Acute pulmonary embolism
C. Hypersensitivity pneumonitis
D. Dyspnea due to obesity
E. Amniotic fluid embolus

92.

A 45-year-old female presents to your office complaining of fever and shortness of breath. This is the 4th Monday in the past 2 months that she has come to see you for this complaint. She began to wheeze and cough this morning, and as the day progressed, she developed fever to 101.5° F and shortness of breath. She bought a parakeet in the last few months.

Meds: HCTZ and lovastatin

PE: T 101.7° F, RR 22, HR 89, BP 136/82.
Mild respiratory distress.
No jugular venous distention.

Lungs show symmetric expansion, normal resonance, diffuse wheezing, and inspiratory crackles audible at the bases.

Remaining exam is normal.

CXR: Diffuse alveolar filling pattern and variable interstitial streaks.

For which of the following is this patient at risk if the correct diagnosis is missed today?

A. Interstitial fibrosis
B. Lymphoma
C. Sudden cardiac death
D. Obstructive lung disease
E. Diffuse alveolar hemorrhage

93.

On a routine x-ray film of the chest, a 62-year-old man has a solitary pulmonary nodule. He has smoked one pack of cigarettes daily for 40 years and has had early-morning cough and expectoration for 5 years. The lesion is 2.4 cm in diameter, peripheral, and contains no calcium deposits on chest CT.

PMH is significant for rheumatoid arthritis for 10 years. Physical examination confirms bilateral metacarpal involvement with bilateral ulnar deviation of the digits. He has rheumatoid nodules over the extensor surface of his right forearm. Laboratory tests show a rheumatoid factor of 1:1280. His tuberculosis skin test was positive 2 years ago, and he completed 9 months of isoniazid. The patient feels well, except for his morning cough.

Which of the following is the <u>most</u> appropriate management?

    A. Advise the patient to stop smoking; perform no additional studies.
    B. Repeat a low-dose helical CT scan in 3 months.
    C. Obtain sputum for mycobacterial culture and acid-fast smear.
    D. Refer for biopsy or surgical removal of the nodule.
    E. Start etanercept.

94.

A 45-year-old hospital orderly complains of progressive shortness of breath with ambulation for 2 weeks. Over the past week, he has also developed a nonproductive cough that is worse at night. He is otherwise healthy and does not smoke or use drugs.

Lung exam: symmetric excursions, decreased resonance to percussion, and reduced tactile fremitus at the left base

CXR: Left pleural effusion

TB skin test: 13 mm
Induced sputum shows no acid-fast organisms
Sputum NAA is pending

Thoracentesis:
pH 7.20
Glucose 67 mg/dL
LDH 1162 IU/L
Protein 6.5 g/dL
Cells 133 cells/mm3
    (30% neutrophils, 60% lymphocytes)
Acid-fast smears show no organisms

Which of the following is the <u>most</u> appropriate next step in patient care?

    A. Intravenous ceftriaxone.
    B. Oral prednisone.
    C. No treatment and follow-up repeat CXR in 6 weeks.
    D. MRI of the chest with thin cuts through the diaphragm.
    E. Start isoniazid, rifampin, pyrazinamide, and ethambutol.

95.

A 27-year-old complains of "chest pain" and fever. He is diagnosed with pneumonia and treated with levofloxacin as an outpatient 10 days ago. At the time he had rust-colored sputum with lancet-shaped, gram-positive diplococci.

Initially he improved, but now on day 4 after starting therapy, he has developed new fever and right-sided, pleuritic chest pain.

A CT scan of the chest is done, and the results are presented here:

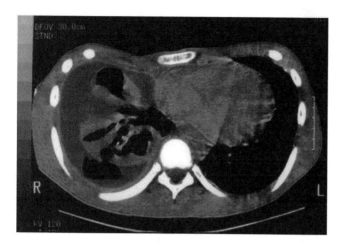

What is the <u>most</u> appropriate next step in management?

A. Add oral amoxicillin-clavulanic acid for anaerobe coverage.
B. Schedule a CT-pulmonary angiogram.
C. Send acid-fast smears and cultures of sputum and place a TB skin test.
D. Attempt tube thoracostomy with CT guidance with possible need for more invasive therapy depending on response.
E. Begin prednisone 60 mg daily with 10-day wean.

CARDIOLOGY

96.

A 65-year-old man complains of chest pain when walking up 5 flights of stairs. The pain is right-sided, sharp in character, lasts a few minutes, and resolves with rest. He has never had a diagnosis of coronary artery disease or MI. He has a history of hypertension and hyperlipidemia; both are well controlled on hydrochlorothiazide and atorvastatin. He is otherwise in good health. He has never smoked cigarettes and does not drink alcohol. Family history is unremarkable. Review of systems is otherwise negative. The physical examination is normal. Baseline electrocardiogram is normal.

Vital Signs: BP: 138/82 mmHg, Pulse: 82 bpm, Respirations: 12, afebrile.

He has a 90% pretest probability of having coronary artery disease.

You order an exercise stress test, and the results return:
"Target heart rate achieved. No ST changes during exercise. No evidence of reperfusion defects."

You have a graph looking at pre/posttest probabilities.

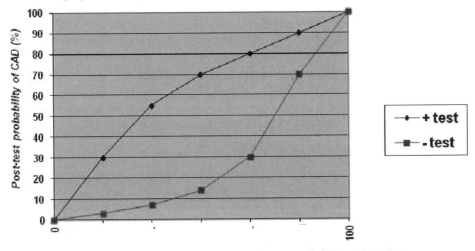

With this test result, how much less likely is this patient to have cardiac artery disease (CAD)?

   A. 50% less likely (30% posttest probability of CAD)
   B. 70% less likely (10% posttest probability of CAD)
   C. 20% less likely (70% posttest probability of CAD)
   D. Below 5% posttest probability of CAD
   E. Unchanged

97.

A 67-year-old man was admitted to the CCU with an acute ST-segment elevation MI. He was stabilized and initially received aspirin, thrombolytic therapy, heparin, nitrates, and beta-blockers. On day 2, he has multiple runs of ventricular tachycardia that are asymptomatic and last only a few seconds. Eventually, his thrombolytics and anticoagulants are discontinued. On day 5, he becomes acutely short of breath.

Vital signs: BP: 96/50 mmHg, pulse: 110 bpm, respiration: 24, afebrile.

On exam, there is a systolic murmur that begins in mid-systole and extends to the second heart sound. It is audible over the entire chest.

Which of the following is the <u>most</u> appropriate next step in patient care?

    A. Re-institute thrombolytic therapy for a recurrent MI.
    B. Immediately aspirate the pericardial sac for presumed tamponade.
    C. Prescribe massive volume resuscitation for presumed right ventricular infarction.
    D. Order an immediate surgical consultation for repair of a ventricular septal defect.
    E. Order an immediate surgical consultation for repair of a ruptured papillary muscle.

98.

You see a 30-year-old man in the emergency department who has been experiencing palpitations for the past 2 hours. He has had similar symptoms in the past, but the symptoms have not lasted as long as this episode. He is otherwise healthy. He takes no medications, has never smoked, drinks alcohol only on weekends, and has never used illicit drugs. There is a family history of premature coronary artery disease (both grandfathers died in their 50s from MI).

On physical exam, he appears nervous, but healthy.
Vital signs: BP: 110/68 mmHg, Pulse: 155 bpm, Respirations: 12, Temperature: Afebrile
The exam is unremarkable except for tachycardia. PMI is nondisplaced, and estimated JVP is 4 mmHg.

An ECG is performed:

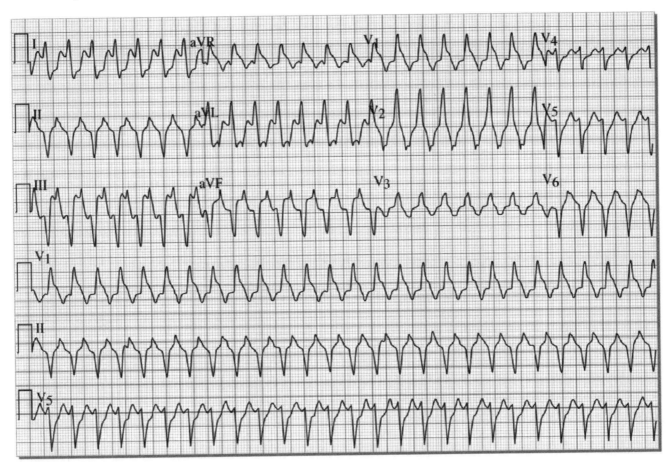

Conscious sedation with synchronized cardioversion is the best treatment if available quickly.

If conscious sedation with synchronized cardioversion is <u>not</u> available, which of the following is the <u>most</u> appropriate next step in the management of this patient?

  A. Metoprolol intravenously
  B. Adenosine intravenously
  C. Verapamil intravenously
  D. Amiodarone intravenously

99.

A 60-year-old man has questions about the safety of his medications. He drinks 2 glasses of grapefruit juice each morning, but recently saw a "20/20" TV show segment on the dangers of grapefruit juice in patients taking "heart medicines." He is currently prescribed benazepril, hydrochlorothiazide, warfarin, omeprazole, simvastatin, and loratadine.

Which of his drugs is affected by grapefruit juice?

    A. Loratadine
    B. Simvastatin
    C. Omeprazole
    D. Warfarin
    E. Benazepril

100.

You are asked to evaluate a 56-year-old woman prior to elective hip replacement for severe osteoarthritis. She is otherwise healthy and takes only intermittent acetaminophen for the pain.

Previous Medical History/Previous Surgical History: None.
Allergies: None.
Review of Systems: She has poor functional capacity because of the osteoarthritis.

Her physical exam is normal, except for decreased range of motion of the hip

Which of the following preoperative tests is indicated?

    A. No testing; send to the operating room.
    B. Basic metabolic panel, CBC, ECG, U/A.
    C. Cardiac function testing (e.g., thallium).
    D. Comprehensive metabolic panel, CBC.
    E. Hematocrit, ECG.

101.

A 72-year-old man with Type 2 DM and a history of MI 6 years ago is found to have a pulsatile abdominal mass on exam. Ultrasound reveals a 7-cm aortic aneurysm. He walks 8–10 blocks every day without symptoms. You are asked to examine this patient and advise on what is needed prior to aortic surgery.

Exam:
BP: 120/70 mmHg
Pulse: 75 bpm
Chest: Clear
Cardiac: Normal S_1 and S_2, no murmur
HCT: 38%
Glu: 160 mg/dL

ECG is as follows:

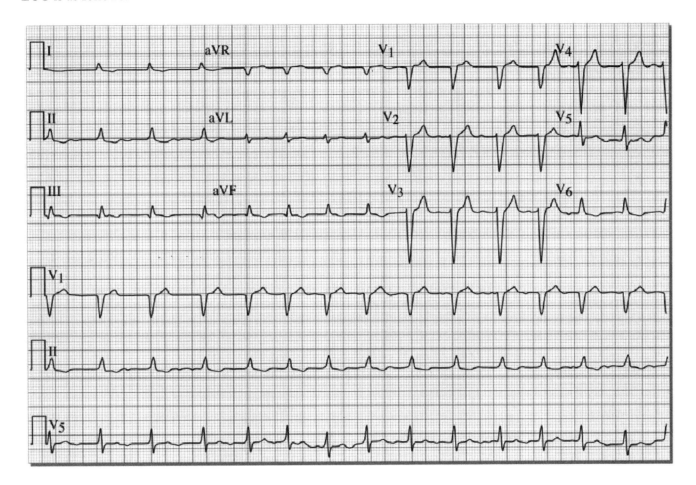

Which of the following would you recommend?

    A. Proceed with surgery,
    B. Obtain TTE before surgery.
    C. Complete a risk assessment with thallium stress test.
    D. Complete a risk assessment with cardiac catheterization.
    E. No surgery.

102.

A 27-year-old woman presents for a routine examination. She reports no health problems and has no significant family history. She does not use drugs, tobacco, or alcohol. She takes no medications. Review of systems is unremarkable.

On exam, her blood pressure is 176/88 mmHg and pulse is 70 bpm. On funduscopic exam, AV nicking is present. A systolic and diastolic bruit over the right side of the abdomen is auscultated. The remainder of the exam is normal.

ECG: Sinus rhythm with no Q waves, no evidence of hypertrophy, and no ST-T wave changes.

Repeat blood pressure in one week is 174/90 mmHg. You begin a workup for secondary causes of hypertension. Her potassium is normal.

Which of the following is most likely to confirm the diagnosis?

A. Evaluation of renal function
B. Evaluation of the adrenal gland with contrast tomography and electrolyte measurements
C. Evaluation of the renal arteries with duplex ultrasound
D. Measurement of vanillylmandelic acid and metanephrines in a 24-hour urine collection
E. Evaluation of the renal arteries with angiography

103.

A 29-year-old woman presents with fatigue and chest discomfort with exertion. Review of systems is negative for syncope, cough, skin rashes, arthritis, fevers, and weight loss. She reports no family history of coronary artery disease.

Physical examination reveals clear lung fields, a systolic lift along the left sternal border, and a normal split S_2 with a loud second component. No cardiac murmur is present.

Chest radiograph is remarkable only for bilateral prominent pulmonary arteries without pulmonary congestion. Spirometry is normal.

Which of the following is the _most_ appropriate next step in diagnosis?

A. Right heart catheterization
B. Open lung biopsy
C. Methacholine challenge test
D. Cardiac stress test
E. Echocardiogram

104.

A 78-year-old man with a history of hypertension and DM falls and fractures his shoulder. He will require shoulder surgery. He lives alone and performs all of his activities of daily living. He has no history of CAD or heart failure. Review of systems is negative for chest pains, orthopnea, paroxysmal nocturnal dyspnea, and lower extremity edema.

Physical examination:
BP: 150/90 mmHg
Pulse: 90 bpm
Chest: Clear
Cardiac: Normal S_1/S_2, +S_4, no murmur
Ext: No edema

Laboratory results:
HB: 11 mg/dL
Hct: 33 %   Glu: 148 mg/dL
ECG: NSR, mild LVH

Which of the following would you recommend?

A. Persantine thallium stress test.
B. Echocardiogram.
C. Transfuse 2 units of blood.
D. Okay for immediate surgery.

105.

A 50-year-old man presents to the emergency department with a history of crescendo-pattern chest pain and is admitted to the CCU. While in the CCU, he develops more chest pain, and the nursing staff records a 12-lead ECG that shows 15-mm ST-segment elevation in leads V3 and V5 with additional lesser elevations in leads I, aVL, and V6. These changes revert to normal almost immediately following the administration of sublingual nitroglycerin.

Based on your clinical and ECG findings, which of the following medications would be contraindicated in this patient?

A. Isosorbide dinitrate
B. Nifedipine
C. Lovastatin
D. Diltiazem
E. Propranolol

106.

A 35-year-old woman with systemic lupus erythematosus complains of fatigue and vague abdominal pain. She has vomited twice today. Her blood pressure during inspiration is 70/40—during expiration it increases to 90/40. Neck vein distension is noted on exam. Heart tones are muffled.

ECG findings would be most likely to include:

A. Bradycardia
B. Low voltage of the QRS complexes
C. Shortened PR interval
D. Prolonged QT interval
E. Complete right bundle-branch block

107.

A 22-year-old female Russian immigrant is hospitalized for evaluation of a swollen, warm and tender ankle and knee. After arrival to her hospital room, she develops fever and an erythematous macular rash associated with pale centers. The rash is located on the trunk and extremities but is not pruritic.

A picture is shown here:

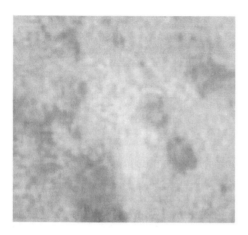

Which of the following results is <u>most</u> likely to be associated with this patient?

A. Elevated antibody titers to *Borrelia burgdorferi*
B. Positive LE cell preparation
C. Blood culture positive for *Salmonella*
D. Prolonged PR interval on ECG
E. Positive culture for *Staphylococcus aureus* following joint aspiration

108.

A 55-year-old man is referred to you for evaluation of a heart murmur, recently heard by your nurse practitioner. On exam, you find that he has a systolic ejection murmur heard best in the right upper sternal border. An ejection click is heard just after S_1. S_2 is muffled. You can make the murmur louder by having him expire or squat.

Which of the following would you expect to find on examination of his carotid artery?

A. Bifid pulse
B. Water-hammer pulse
C. Slowed carotid upstroke
D. Thready pulse
E. Giant right-sided *a* waves

109.

A 32-year-old woman presents with feelings of "doom" and a rapid heartbeat. She has been healthy and without problems until this presentation. On further questioning, however, you discern that she has lost 15 lbs without change in her diet. You also note that she appears to have "bulging" eyes and a fine tremor in her left hand.

An ECG is performed:

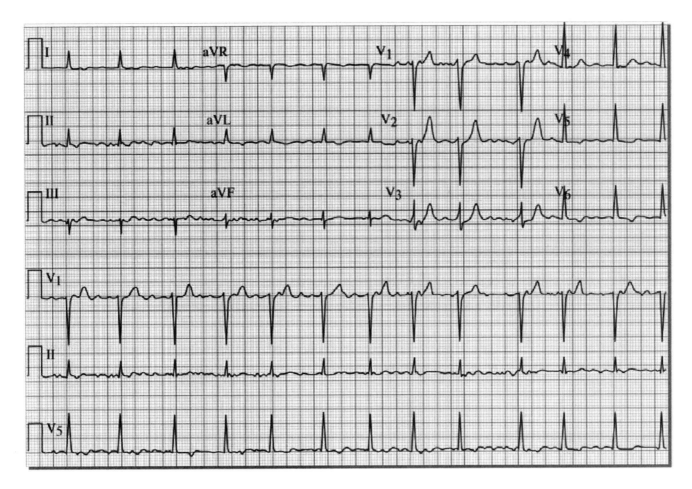

What are you most concerned about at this point?

- A. Eisenmenger transformation
- B. Cor pulmonale
- C. Systemic embolization
- D. Ventricular tachycardia
- E. Bacterial endocarditis

110.

A 54-year-old man presents to the emergency department after a motor vehicle accident. The trauma team notes a heart rate of 150, respiratory rate of 26, and a BP of 80/65 mmHg.

An ECG is quickly done and shows the following:

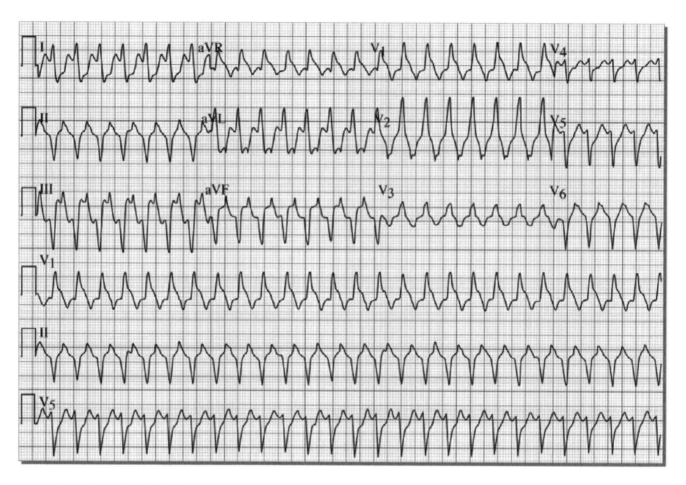

Which of the following is the <u>most</u> appropriate therapy?

- A. IV procainamide
- B. IV dopamine
- C. IV epinephrine
- D. Electrical cardioversion
- E. Pacemaker placement for overdrive pacing

111.

A 23-year-old man is referred to you for evaluation of a heart murmur that was found after an episode of ventricular tachycardia. He also has noted to have "fleeting" chest pains. Your cardiac examination shows a regular rate and rhythm with a normal sounding S_1 and S_2. You note an S_4 as well. He has a systolic ejection murmur, which has the following characteristics: It increases with standing and decreases with a sustained handgrip. Palpation of his chest reveals a "double tap" over the cardiac apex.

Which of the following agents could be used for therapy?

A. Sustained release nitrates
B. Diuretics
C. Fluid restriction and volume depletion
D. Amiodarone
E. Anticoagulants

112.

A 39-year-old woman presents with 2 weeks of dyspnea at rest, orthopnea, and paroxysmal nocturnal dyspnea. She was previously well with no significant past medical history. She uses no prescription medications and has no known drug allergies. She denies a history of upper respiratory infection or use of illicit drugs or cigarettes.

Physical Examination:
She is sitting upright in mild respiratory distress.
HR 120 and regular; BP 100/60; RR 22; Temperature is 37.5° C
JVD: 8 cm
Lungs: Symmetric expansion, resonant to percussion, fine crackles to mid-lung fields bilaterally
Heart: RRR with non-displaced PMI, S_1 slightly diminished, A_2 and P_2 components of S_2 are normal. A 2/6 regurgitant murmur is heard at the left upper sternal border. An S_3 and S_4 are audible at the apex.
Abd: Soft, nontender with mildly tender right upper quadrant and liver span of 11 cm. Hepatojugular reflux is present.
Ext: Trace pedal edema

ECG: Sinus tachycardia with RBBB
CXR: Pulmonary venous congestion with no focal infiltrates

Serum ferritin: 200 ng/mL

Echo: Global decrease in left ventricular systolic function and estimated EF of 25%. Mild mitral and tricuspid regurgitation and no evidence of significant valvular stenosis or intracardiac shunts.

Which of the following is the next __most__ appropriate therapy?

A. Refer for urgent endomyocardial biopsy.
B. Admit to a monitored bed, order iron studies to rule out hemochromatosis.
C. Heart transplant consultation.
D. Admit to the ICU and start intravenous furosemide and an ACE inhibitor.
E. Admit to the ICU and start azathioprine or cyclosporine.

113.

A 43-year-old woman presents to the emergency department with malaise, arthralgias, and a skin rash. She has had a progressive weakness for the past week. Today she is extremely weak. She has no prior significant medical history.

Physical examination:
Temperature is 99.5° F, Pulse 80, RR 30, BP 130/80.
In general she is weak, pale, and ill appearing.
Her skin exam is notable for diffuse, irregular lesions of about 5 mm in size. Some of the lesions are palpable and purpuric, while others are ulcerative.
She has moderate jugular venous distention. Her heart sounds are normal except markedly decreased in intensity. Her lung sounds are clear. She has 1+ pedal edema. Neurologic exam is normal except she is very somnolent, but easily aroused. She falls asleep in mid-sentence.

CXR: Pulmonary vascular congestion
ECG is normal except for notable decrease in amplitude of the QRS complexes.
Sodium 132 mg/dL
Potassium 5 mg/dL
CO_2 19 mEq/L
BUN 105 mg/dL
Creatinine 8.0 mg/dL
Urinalysis shows hematuria with free red blood cells as well as RBC and WBC casts. She has 2+ proteinuria.

Which of the following is the next <u>most</u> appropriate step in diagnosis?

    A. p-ANCA
    B. Echocardiogram
    C. Bilateral lower extremity Doppler ultrasound
    D. ANA, anti-dsDNA
    E. Ventilation/perfusion lung scan

114.

A 61-year-old woman presents to the ER with increasing dyspnea on exertion, shortness of breath at rest, and increasing fatigue. She also has noted new lower extremity edema. She has a known heart murmur since childhood and had an episode of atrial fibrillation at age 45 that resolved spontaneously. Her symptoms have been progressive for about 5–6 months.

Physical Examination:
Afebrile, RR 35, HR 100 and regular, BP 120/66

Significant findings:

Lung exam: Crackles in both bases.

Heart exam: Right ventricular lift is noted. S_1 is normal. S_2 is widely split and fixed with a slightly increased pulmonary component. She has a 2/6 systolic murmur at the left to mid-left upper sternal border. She also has a low-pitched diastolic murmur along the right to mid-right lower sternal border.

Her liver is palpable 4 cm below the right costal margin, and she has 2–3+ peripheral edema.

CXR: Cardiomegaly with prominent main pulmonary artery and increased pulmonary vascularity bilaterally. Her right ventricle appears to be enlarged.

An ECG shows the following:

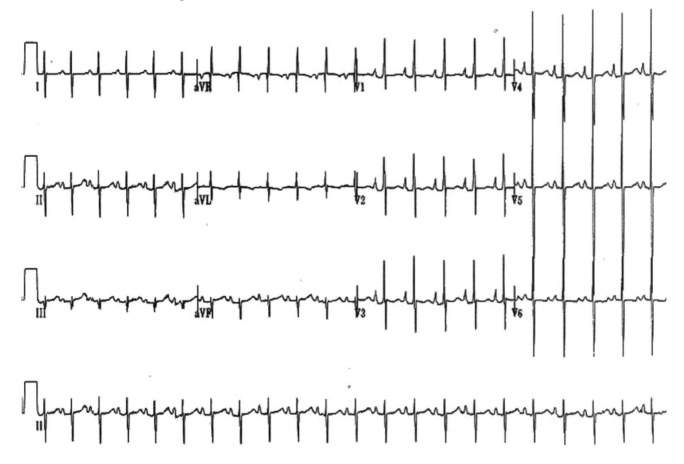

Which of the following is the <u>most</u> likely diagnosis?

    A. Coarctation of the aorta
    B. Tetralogy of Fallot
    C. Ventricular septal defect
    D. Atrial septal defect
    E. Truncus arteriosus

115.

A 33-year-old man presents with increasing shortness of breath and dyspnea on exertion. He says he had a heart murmur as a child but never had it evaluated.

Physical Examination:
He is acyanotic and in no distress at rest.
He is afebrile and has a heart rate of 90, BP is 120/70, and RR is 26.
His chest is clear to auscultation.

His heart exam shows a right ventricular lift. S_1 is normal and S_2 is split with a decreased pulmonary component. There is a systolic click at the left upper sternal border. He has a 3/6 systolic murmur at the left upper sternal border as well. No diastolic murmur is present.

CXR: Mild right ventricular enlargement with post-stenotic dilatation of the main pulmonary artery and normal peripheral pulmonary arteries and lung fields.

ECG shows RAD and RVH.

An echocardiogram is ordered.

Which of the following is the <u>most</u> likely diagnosis?

    A. Coarctation of the aorta
    B. Aortic valve stenosis (AS)
    C. Ventricular septal defect (VSD)
    D. Atrial septal defect (ASD)
    E. Pulmonic valve stenosis (PS)

116.

Your next clinic patient is a 56-year-old man who presents for an insurance physical examination. He has been healthy and reports no health problems. His insurance company requires an ECG, which you perform.

The ECG shows the following:

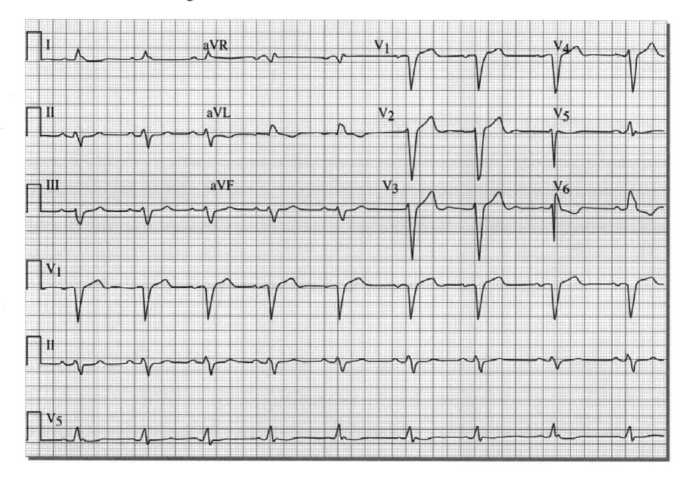

Which of the following does his ECG reveal?

A. Right bundle-branch block (RBBB)
B. Left bundle-branch block (LBBB)
C. 1st degree AV block
D. 2nd degree AV block, Mobitz 1
E. 3rd degree AV block

117.

In a patient with cardiac involvement related to Lyme disease, the __most__ common abnormality is:

A. Coronary artery inflammation
B. Mitral and aortic valve dysfunction
C. Atrioventricular conduction defects
D. Pericardial inflammation

118.

You see a 63-year-old man in the emergency department with long-standing hypertension and hyperlipidemia for chest pain. He is an 80-pack-year smoker. One year ago, he underwent cardiac catheterization because of exertional pain; at that time, he was noted to have 3-vessel coronary artery disease, normal valves, and a normal ejection fraction. His CAD was not amenable to percutaneous coronary intervention (PCI) or CABG. At that time, medical management with a beta-blocker, ASA, and a statin was begun. His exertional chest pain completely resolved.

Today, he describes his pain as severe centrally, radiating to his left arm and back without shortness of breath. He has no other symptoms. This pain was acute and not associated with any sort of exertional pain or shortness of breath prior to today.

On exam, his blood pressure is 180/110 mmHg, pulse 90 bpm, respirations 14, and he is afebrile. There is no elevation of jugular venous pulsations, no S_3, and no rales. You hear a grade II/VI decrescendo murmur in the third left interspace after the second heart sound. There is no edema.

ECG shows 3-mm ST-segment elevations in leads I, aVL, and V2 through V5, and reciprocal ST depressions in leads II and III.

Cardiac troponins are elevated to three times the upper limit of normal.

Which of the following is the next appropriate step in the management of this patient?

A. Pericardiocentesis
B. High-dose ibuprofen
C. Thrombolytic therapy
D. Immediate bedside transesophageal echocardiogram
E. Upper endoscopy

119.

You see a 64-year-old woman with long-standing hypertension, mild renal insufficiency, insulin-requiring diabetes, and a cerebrovascular accident two years ago with residual dysphasia for a preoperative evaluation prior to hip replacement surgery for severe osteoarthritis. Since her stroke, she has had no further cerebrovascular or cardiovascular problems, and has been able to do her usual activities of daily living without chest pain or shortness of breath. She had a nuclear stress-perfusion cardiac stress test one year ago, which was negative for reversible ischemia. She has no other medical history and has never had major surgery.

She takes long-acting insulin daily, with rapid acting insulin at meals; daily aspirin; and hydrochlorothiazide 25 mg daily.

Her blood glucose levels typically range from 90 mg/dL (fasting) to 165 mg/dL after meals.

On exam, her blood pressure is 138/82 mmHg, pulse 80 bpm, respirations 12/min, and she is afebrile. There is no elevation of jugular venous pulsations, no S_3, no murmur, and no rales. There is no edema.

ECG is sinus, with normal intervals and no ST segment or T wave abnormalities.

Chemistry panel shows normal electrolytes, a BUN of 24 mg/dL, and creatinine of 2.2 mg/dL, which is at her baseline. Hemoglobin is 11.2 g/dL. Glycohemoglobin is 6.4%.

Which of the following interventions is <u>most</u> likely to reduce her risk of perioperative cardiovascular complications?

    A. Coronary angiography with percutaneous coronary intervention of stenotic lesions
    B. Perioperative beta-blocker therapy
    C. Preoperative transfusion of packed red blood cells
    D. Preoperative ACE inhibitor therapy
    E. No new intervention

120.

A 57-year-old woman is evaluated for chest pain and taken to the cardiac catheterization lab for evaluation.

She undergoes left heart catheterization, which shows normal coronary arteries and the following pressure tracing:

Left Heart Catheterization Pressure Tracing

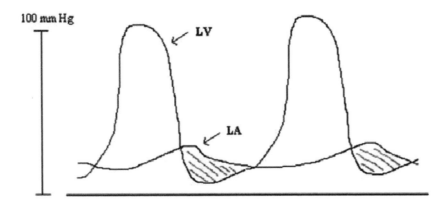

Upon further questioning and examination of this patient, which of the following clinical scenarios is <u>most</u> likely?

   A. A history of multiple syncopal episodes, a crescendo-decrescendo systolic murmur at the base of the heart
   B. A history of untreated strep throat, hemoptysis, and a diastolic rumble at the left 5th interspace at the mid-clavicular line
   C. Exertional dyspnea and a holosystolic murmur at the lower left sternal border
   D. Repeated hospital admissions for CHF, a loud holosystolic murmur, a positive bubble study
   E. A history of IV drug use, positive blood cultures, fever, Osler nodes

121.

You see a 49-year-old man in the emergency department for 30 minutes of crushing substernal chest pain. He has poorly controlled hypertension and a family history of premature coronary artery disease. He takes only HCTZ 25 mg daily and has no other medical problems.

Vital signs are as follows: BP: 158/92 mmHg, pulse: 106, resp: 18, afebrile
His exam is normal, with no evidence of congestive heart failure or murmurs.

ECG shows 2- to 3-mm ST-segment depressions in leads I and aVL and leads V2 through V5. Initial CK is normal, but cardiac troponins are 3x normal.

Cardiology is contacted and plans to take him to the cardiac catheterization lab within the next hour for delineation of his coronary anatomy and probable percutaneous coronary intervention (PCI).

In addition to immediate aspirin and bivalirudin therapy, which of the following is the best treatment option prior to sending the patient for angiography/PCI?

   A. Thrombolytic therapy
   B. Ticagrelor (P2Y12 receptor blocker)
   C. Immediate release nifedipine
   D. No other treatment prior to coronary angiography

122.

A 38-year-old woman with recurrent hematuria is scheduled for cystoscopy. She is otherwise healthy, has never had surgery, takes no medications, does not smoke cigarettes, drink alcohol, or use IV drugs. Review of systems is negative.

Physical exam is normal, except for a sharp, short sound heard in mid-systole followed by a Grade II/VI murmur audible at the apex.

What antibiotic prophylaxis for infective endocarditis should be given to this patient?

   A. One dose of oral amoxicillin prior to the procedure
   B. Intravenous ceftriaxone
   C. Intravenous ampicillin plus gentamicin perioperatively
   D. None of the choices

123.

An unidentified male, in his 30s, is recovered after falling through the ice at the local park. He is believed to have been submerged for 20–30 minutes. EMS was called and found him in asystole. Emergency resuscitation was instituted. The patient was intubated; CPR was continued, and he was brought to the local emergency department.

On physical examination, there is no pulse, no spontaneous respirations, and his core body temperature is 80° F (26.7° C). Cardiac compressions and external ventilation have been in progress for 20 minutes without spontaneous resumption of cardiac conduction or respirations.

What is the best next appropriate step in the treatment of this patient?

  A. Due to the extended period of non-responsiveness, pronounce the patient dead.
  B. Aggressively treat the hypothermia and continue with resuscitation efforts until core temperature is > 33° C (91.4° F).
  C. Obtain an urgent neurology consultation to assist with a brain death evaluation.
  D. Transfer the body to the operating room in preparation for organ harvest.

124.

Brain natriuretic peptide (BNP) is a hormone released from cardiac tissue that acts on receptors in the kidneys, smooth muscles of the blood vessels, and the adrenal glands. The overall effect is to increase urine production and sodium excretion, reduce vascular resistance, and diminish the release of renin and aldosterone.

For which of the following situations is measurement of BNP <u>most</u> useful?

  A. A patient with elevated JVP, pulmonary congestion, peripheral edema, and an S_3 on auscultation
  B. A patient with chronic COPD, basilar crepitus, and pedal edema presenting with increased shortness of breath and the etiology of the worsening symptoms is in question
  C. A patient with a transient ischemic attack, a right-sided carotid bruit, and a history of hyperlipidemia
  D. A patient with hypertension, a renal bruit, and evidence of fluid retention

125.

You begin evaluation of a 27-year-old male who presented to the emergency department with severe chest pain that started abruptly 3 hours previously. The pain was in the anterior central chest and lasted for 1–2 hours. He experienced light-headedness but no diaphoresis. The pain has currently improved to a moderate ache.

On examination, the patient is distressed and appears to be mildly uncomfortable. He is wearing glasses secondary to a lens displacement that is being followed by ophthalmology. His heart rate is 94/min, respiratory rate is 12 breaths/min, and blood pressure is 142/88 mmHg. The patient is afebrile. His height is 6' 6" (198.1 cm), and he weighs 157 lbs (71.4 kg). Exam of the chest reveals moderate pectus excavatum. He has a regular rhythm and is noted to have a soft systolic murmur at the apex with a late systolic click. Lungs are clear with good air entry. No JVD is present. Peripheral pulses are present. There is no swelling or tenderness in the extremities.

There is widening of the mediastinum noted on an x-ray of the chest.

ECG demonstrates no acute changes or dysrhythmias.

Which of the following is the **most** likely etiology of this person's chest pain?

A. Acute myocardial infarction (MI)
B. Acute pericarditis
C. Mitral valve prolapse (MVP)
D. Aortic dissection
E. Pulmonary embolism (PE)

126.

A 23-year-old male migrant worker presents to the emergency department with complaints of shortness of breath and fatigue. The symptoms have been progressively worse over the last 2–3 years, but he has deferred seeking medical help due to difficulties with his immigration status.

On examination, the patient is dyspneic at rest without labored breathing. His lungs are clear with good air entry. There is mild elevation in the JVP and a jugular venous pulse wave is noted. Cardiac exam demonstrates a normal S_1 with a loud pulmonary component of the second heart sound and a regular rhythm. There is a soft systolic murmur at the left sternal border. Palpation of the chest reveals a right ventricular heave. Pulses in the extremities are present. There is cyanosis of the toes, but not of the fingers. Clubbing is noted.

Right ventricular strain pattern was evident on electrocardiogram.

Enlarged pulmonary arteries with no infiltrates were noted on chest radiography. Cardiac silhouette is suggestive of right atrial and right ventricular hypertrophy.

Which of the following is **most** likely to be found on cardiac catheterization?

A. Ventricular septal defect (VSD)
B. Patent ductus arteriosus (PDA)
C. Pulmonic stenosis (PS)
D. Aortic stenosis (AS)

127.

In an adult, which of the following conditions would **most** likely benefit from prophylactic antibiotics to prevent endocarditis?

A. Previous coronary artery bypass graft (CABG) surgery.
B. Isolated ostium secundum atrial septal defect (ASD).
C. Implanted cardiac defibrillator.
D. Effective surgical repair of a ventricular septal defect (VSD) in childhood.
E. None of the choices would benefit.

128.

A 35-year-old female comes with several family members to your clinic to discuss results from a recent out-of-area hospitalization. She was visiting family at that time and was prompted to visit the area's emergency department when she experienced chest pain. She was admitted at that time for evaluation. During her workup, cardiac enzymes were normal; exercise tolerance testing demonstrated no abnormalities, and an echocardiogram was remarkable only for mitral valve prolapse (MVP) without regurgitation or valvular thickening. She was discharged on a beta-blocker.

The patient now wants your opinion as to the long-term prognosis of her condition.

Which of the following would you tell her about her MVP?

    A. It increases her risk for sudden death.
    B. Left ventricular failure is a common consequence.
    C. Her current condition is benign.
    D. She should receive antibiotics before dental procedures.
    E. It increases her risk of systemic emboli.

129.

An ECG for a 43-year-old female demonstrates the following rhythm:

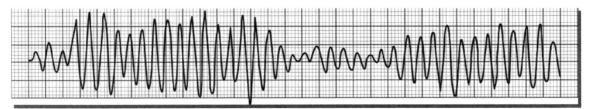

Which of the following electrolyte abnormalities is <u>most</u> likely to cause this rhythm?

    A. Hyperkalemia
    B. Hypomagnesemia
    C. Hypocalcemia
    D. Hypernatremia

130.

A 34-year-old female presents to the clinic with complaints of pain and swelling in her right leg that has been worsening over the previous 24 hours. She is markedly obese. She has no previous history of deep venous thrombosis.

D-dimer measurement would be <u>most</u> helpful in association with which of the following conditions?

    A. A high probability ventilation-perfusion scan
    B. No swelling or signs of inflammation on right leg exam
    C. Doppler exam demonstrating a right leg deep venous thrombosis
    D. Second trimester of pregnancy

131.

A 63-year-old female who has been a patient in your clinic for many years returns for ongoing evaluation related to complaints of shortness of breath, which has been developing over several months. One week previously, you started an evaluation for symptoms and findings of congestive heart failure. Initial lab work was obtained, and the patient was scheduled for echocardiography.

Remarkable among the results were significant protein in her urine and mild elevations of BUN and creatinine.

Her chest x-ray showed an increase in the cardiothoracic ratio, with mildly increased pulmonary vasculature. No infiltrates were reported.

Echocardiogram report noted no pericardial effusion, near-normal intraventricular dimensions, symmetric biventricular thickening, hypokinesis, and diffuse "granular sparkling."

On examination, the patient is in no marked distress at rest. She has a small amount of petechiae around the eyes bilaterally, and there is a general fullness to the tongue. She has mild basilar rales that improve but do not resolve with deep breathing. Cardiac exam demonstrates a regular rate and rhythm without rub, gallop, or murmur. The abdomen is benign, and a normal liver span is noted. There is a mild amount of pitting edema bilaterally. No other prominent skin lesions or discolorations are noted. Neurologic examination was within normal limits.

Which of the following is most likely to be the cause of this patient's cardiac condition?

A. Amyloidosis
B. Fabry disease
C. Hemochromatosis
D. Sarcoidosis

132.

A 56-year-old male presents to your clinic with complaints of generalized fatigue and palpitations. Over the last eight weeks, he has experienced headache, malaise, myalgias, and increasing fatigue. He was doing well prior to this time.

He is semi-retired and spends his summers in northern Wisconsin and his winters in Texas. He has been working around his wooded property in Wisconsin over the last 3 months. He has no known exposures to persons with an infection or to other illnesses. He did note a rash that started as a non-itchy patch in the right groin that slowly spread to the upper right thigh. He started treatment with over-the-counter antifungal cream. There was central clearing initially, but some redness recurred in the center. After three weeks of antifungal cream, the rash eventually resolved.

The patient is noted to have an irregular rhythm, and an ECG is obtained:

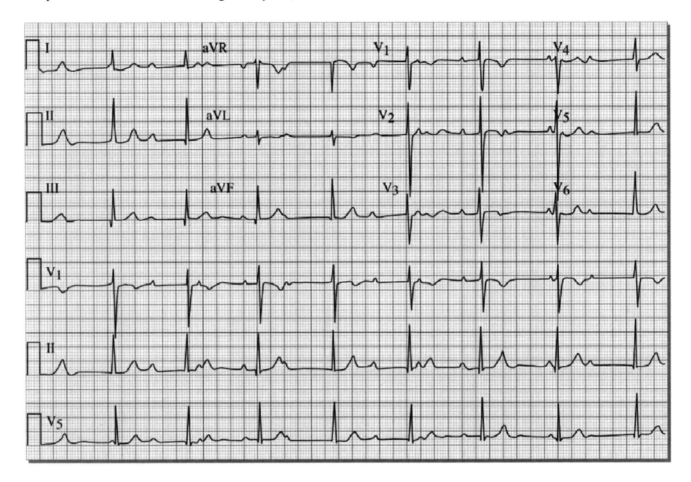

Which of the following is the <u>most</u> appropriate next step in patient care?

   A. Long-term pacemaker intervention
   B. Intravenous ceftriaxone and possible temporary pacing
   C. Prescription of aspirin because this patient has a long-term risk of coronary artery aneurysm
   D. Oral cephalexin

133.

A 29-year-old female cocaine abuser is seen in the emergency department with complaints of chest pain following a binge of cocaine usage.

Which of the following should <u>not</u> be used for initial treatment?

   A. Calcium channel blockers
   B. Beta-blockers
   C. Benzodiazepines
   D. Nitroglycerin

134.

You are asked to counsel an 18-year-old freshman in the college health center. He comes with a tracing from his local physician who has asked him not to participate in sports without consultation with a physician at the college.

Here is his tracing:

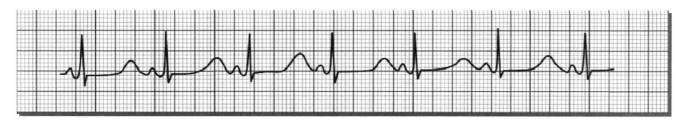

He is very interested in participating in intramural sports and wants advice as to which sport would be the safest to participate.

Which of the following sports poses the lowest risk for the patient?

    A. Diving
    B. Soccer
    C. Golf
    D. Basketball
    E. Swimming

135.

A 54-year-old post-menopausal female presents with intermittent chest pain. The pain occurs with exercise and causes shortness of breath, aching pain in the left shoulder, and some palpitations. It resolves in 15–20 minutes with rest. She has no history of diabetes mellitus or hypertension. Her LMP was 6 years previously. She smokes 4–5 cigarettes/day.

She undergoes exercise-tolerance testing and experiences an episode of pain similar to her original complaints. Her blood pressure is within expected ranges, and ST depression in the anteroseptal leads is noted. There is marginal response to sublingual nitroglycerin, but the pain and ST changes resolve with rest. She then undergoes cardiac catheterization that reveals normal coronary arteries.

What is the __most__ appropriate next step in her evaluation?

    A. There is no definite test for diagnosis, and it is a diagnosis of exclusion.
    B. Electrophysiological studies (EPS).
    C. Psychiatric referral.
    D. Upper endoscopy with manometry.
    E. Urine studies for catecholamines.

136.

You receive the report of an electrophysiologic study (EPS), which was performed for a 35-year-old male. This patient has been seen in the emergency department multiple times for symptomatic tachycardia, and subsequent evaluation included an EPS. The report documents an accessory pathway and indicates a propensity for the conduction to be antegrade down the accessory pathway and retrograde in the normal pathway. The patient strongly desires a resolution to the problem but has been exceptionally nonadherent to medications and follow-up in the recent past.

Which of the following is the best intervention to resolve his current cardiac issue?

A. Surgical ablation of the accessory pathway
B. Radiofrequency ablation of the accessory pathway
C. Long-term digitalis treatment
D. Long-term propranolol treatment
E. Placement of a chronic pacemaker

137.

Erectile dysfunction is often associated with cardiovascular processes. Newer interventions, including medications, are being developed to improve erectile function. Among these are medications such as sildenafil (Viagra®), tadalafil (Cialis®), avanafil (Stendra®) and vardenafil (Levitra®, Staxyn®).

Which of the following conditions is <u>most</u> likely to result in an adverse event when one of these agents is administered?

A. Atrial fibrillation and warfarin
B. Mitral valve prolapse and propranolol
C. Angina and isosorbide dinitrate
D. Congestive heart failure and digitalis
E. Hypertrophic cardiomyopathy and verapamil

138.

You are called to admit a 32-year-old male who presented to the emergency department with complaints of chest pain. He is admitted to a monitored floor and, during the course of hospitalization, he is shown to have experienced a myocardial infarction. A homocysteine level is found to be very high.

Which of the following is <u>not</u> routinely included in the treatment of an acute MI in this young patient?

A. Beta-blockers
B. Statins
C. Aspirin
D. B vitamin supplements
E. ACE inhibitors

139.

A 54-year-old male, who works as a postal carrier, presents to the clinic with complaints of bilateral lower leg pain. He normally drives a delivery truck on his mail route, but occasionally must walk to deliver items. He has noted pain in the lower legs. It occurs at about 200 meters of walking or after climbing two flights of stairs. The cramping pain improves after 3–5 minutes of rest, and then he can resume activity. He is a social drinker and smokes 1 pack/day. He denies any illicit drugs.

On physical examination, there is significant difficulty palpating the dorsalis pedis and posterior tibialis pulses bilaterally. The capillary refill of the nail beds on the feet is mildly delayed.

Which is the <u>most</u> appropriate next intervention?

    A. Refer for lower extremity angiography.
    B. Advise patient to restrict activity as much as possible.
    C. Smoking cessation.
    D. Prescribe support stockings.
    E. Institute dipyridamole therapy.

140.

Which of the following conditions is <u>most</u> appropriate for pharmacologic (non-exercise) stress testing?

    A. Severe claudication
    B. Digitalis therapy
    C. Cardiac pacemaker
    D. Diabetes mellitus

141.

A 65-year-old man presents in the emergency department with a 10-minute history of severe crushing chest pain. He describes the pain as a "horse sitting on my chest." Nitroglycerin given by paramedics temporarily relieved the pain. He presents now as an anxious man in no apparent distress. His pain occurred 1 hour ago, and he arrived in the emergency department 20 minutes ago. He had a normal ECG last year.

His current ECG is shown here:

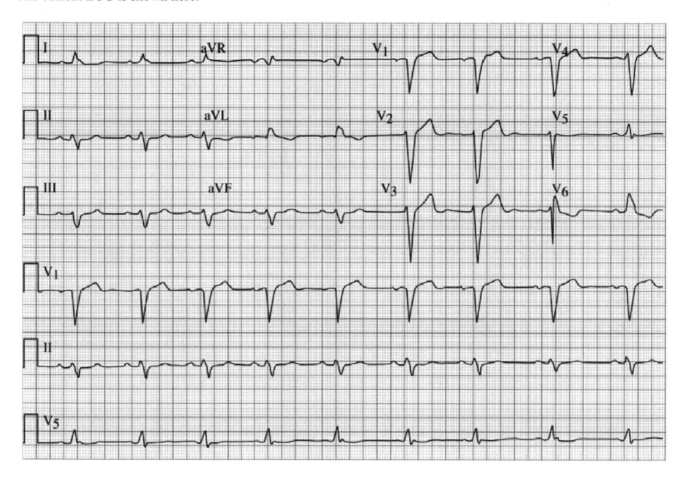

Initial cardiac enzymes are abnormal.

What is the best therapy for this patient?

A. Monitor his rhythm for 12 hours and if stable, schedule for stress echo.
B. Do not give fibrinolytics, because he has a posterior MI.
C. Give fibrinolytic therapy if not contraindicated and if primary percutaneous coronary intervention is not immediately available.
D. Immediately perform a stress study to provoke ischemia, and evaluate LV function via ECHO if ischemia is present.
E. Because he has only minor ST elevation, it is reasonable to admit him to the CCU and observe for 24 hours.

142.

You see a 65-year-old female patient, who is new to your practice. She tells you that her old doctor mentioned "something about aortic stenosis," but she did not fully understand and didn't ask any questions. Now she is concerned, although she reports no chest pain, weakness, or palpitations. Her exam is normal.

Which of the following is <u>most</u> consistent with the diagnosis of aortic stenosis?

A. It is not a common congenital cardiac anomaly.
B. Patients with bicuspid aortic valves develop aortic stenosis two decades later than patients with trileaflet valves.
C. Once symptoms develop with aortic stenosis, prognosis is poor.
D. Sudden death occurs in < 1% of patients, almost all of whom are symptomatic.
E. A systolic thrill, if it occurs, is located in the right axilla.

143.

The phenomenon of *torsades de pointes* in its pure form is best viewed in conjunction with prolongation of which of the following interval measurements?

A. PR interval
B. QRS duration
C. QTc interval
D. R-R interval
E. QP interval

144.

You are called to the emergency department to see a 31-year-old woman who noticed a sudden erratic beating of her heart and became "sweaty." On further questioning, you learn that she has lost 10 pounds without change in her diet. You notice slightly bulging eyes, a fine tremor, and her pulse is abnormally irregular.

A tracing is as follows:

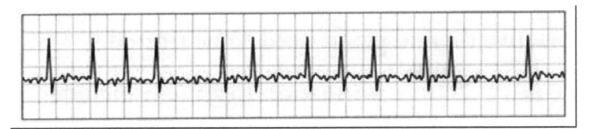

You now are anxious to restore sinus rhythm because of the cumulative risk of which of the following?

A. Eisenmenger transformation
B. Bacterial endocarditis
C. Cor pulmonale
D. Systemic embolization
E. Pulmonary thromboembolism

145.

A 30-year-old woman with no past medical history presents complaining of 6 months of shortness of breath and fatigue. She first noticed something was wrong when she began to experience episodic painful swelling in her ankles and hands that spontaneously resolved. She has noticed a severe reduction in her ability to perform her daily routine. She now has to rest while dressing herself in the mornings. The last episode of joint swelling lasted for 2 weeks and occurred 3 months ago. Review of systems is positive for a mild nonproductive cough, increasing bilateral lower extremity edema, 25-pound weight loss over 1 year, alopecia, 3 spontaneous abortions, and Raynaud phenomenon. Review of systems is negative for orthopnea, paroxysmal nocturnal dyspnea, unilateral leg swellings, and snoring. Family history is positive for maternal hypertension. She takes no medications and denies drug use or excessive alcohol intake.

Physical exam reveals a normal radial pulse, a loud P_2 component of the 2nd heart sound, and normal lung sounds. Edema is present in both feet.

Which of the following findings is also likely to be present?

    A. Prominent *a* and *v* waves with hepatomegaly
    B. Normal jugular venous pulsations
    C. Equal *a* and *v* waves with a low-voltage electrocardiogram
    D. Giant *a* waves with a blunted *y* descent
    E. Irregular cannon *a* waves

146.

A 45-year-old woman presents with acute shortness of breath and chest pain. She has a recent history of breast cancer and began chemotherapy 2 weeks ago. Her BP is 70/50 mmHg. She is admitted to the ICU and undergoes right heart catheterization. Noted are the following findings: RA pressure is 18 mmHg; PA pressure is 34/18 mmHg; PCWP is 17 mmHg; and her BP remains low at 70/48 mmHg.

Based on these findings, which of the following is <u>most</u> likely occurring?

    A. Cardiogenic shock
    B. RV infarction
    C. Pulmonary hypertension
    D. Tamponade
    E. Mitral stenosis

147.

A 35-year-old woman presents with sudden onset of shortness of breath. She has atrial fibrillation on the monitor. The physical examination shows an opening snap at the apex, and the S_1 appears to be loud. You hear a low-pitched diastolic rumble at the apex. ECG shows atrial fibrillation with left atrial enlargement.

Which of the following cardiac abnormalities is <u>most</u> likely?

A. Mitral regurgitation
B. Aortic regurgitation
C. Mitral stenosis
D. Aortic stenosis
E. Hypertrophic cardiomyopathy

148.

A 45-year-old man presents with severe chest pain. He has fever and is tachycardic. The pain is relieved by sitting forward. You perform an ECG:

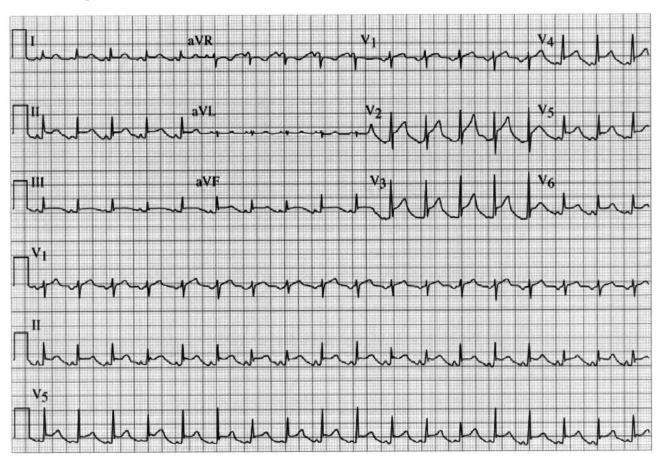

Which of the following is the <u>most</u> likely diagnosis?

A. Acute pericarditis
B. Acute tamponade
C. Acute pneumonia
D. Acute left ventricular MI
E. Acute cardiogenic shock

149.

A 70-year-old woman presents with acute shortness of breath and chest discomfort. She has a history of angina, has been on beta-blockers, and intermittently takes nitroglycerin tablets when she experiences exertional chest pain.

Her ECG:

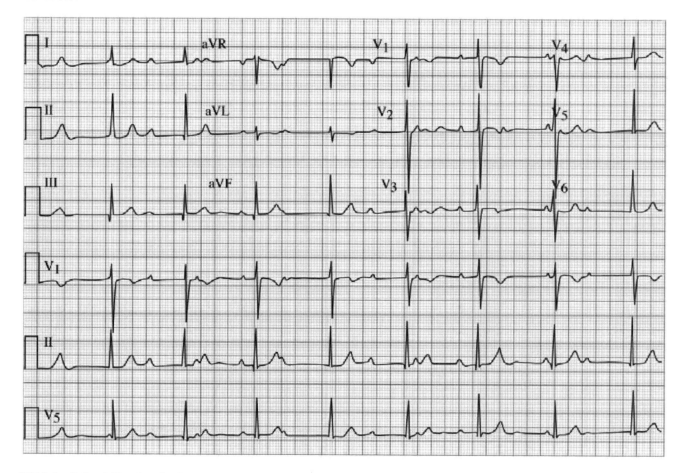

Which of the following is the <u>most</u> appropriate next step?

A. Stop beta-blockers because this shows an allergic reaction.
B. Initiate pacing because this is 3rd degree AV block.
C. Initiate pacing because this is symptomatic 2nd degree AV block.
D. No pacing is indicated because this is 1st degree AV block.

150.

A 31-year-old woman presents for a pre-employment physical. Her ECG:

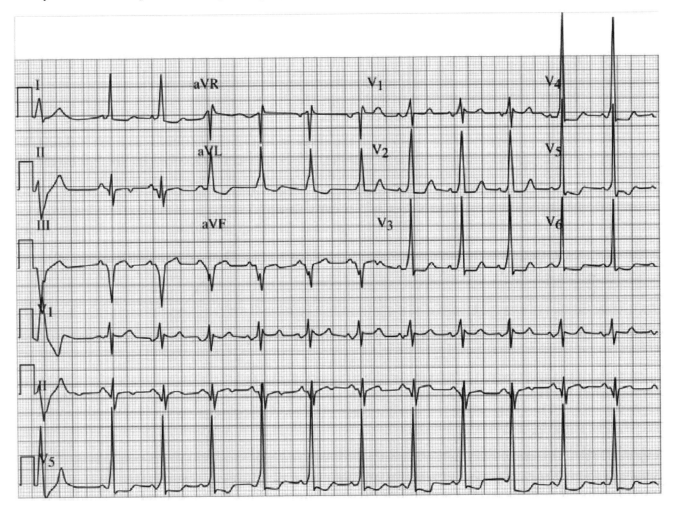

What does the ECG show?

A. 2nd degree AV block, type 1
B. 2nd degree AV block, type 2
C. 3rd degree AV block
D. Wolff-Parkinson-White syndrome (WPW)
E. Acute pericarditis

151.

A 28-year-old woman with diabetes presents in septic shock and develops cardiac arrhythmias. On further questioning, her husband notes that she is 20 weeks pregnant. She had been doing well until this morning when she suddenly felt ill and began vomiting. Soon afterward, she developed fever. Blood cultures are pending. She is intubated and continues to have various arrhythmias with hypotension. She also appears to have congestive heart failure.

Which of the following is contraindicated?

A. Elective electrical cardioversion
B. Procainamide
C. Digoxin
D. Enalapril
E. Verapamil

152.

A 26-year-old woman presents to the emergency department after fainting. An ECG shows a long QT interval. She admits that she had been staying up late for several weeks working and has spent long hours in the hot tub to relax. The day before fainting, she was told that she might be laid off of her job, and she panicked.

Which of the following would __most__ likely prolong her QT interval?

A. Hypercalcemia
B. Tricyclic overdose
C. Hypermagnesemia
D. Hyperkalemia
E. Low-fat diet

153.

A 67-year-old man with Type 2 DM and history of myocardial infarction 6 years ago is found to have a pulsatile abdominal mass on exam. Ultrasound reveals a 7-cm aortic aneurysm that requires surgery. He walks 8–10 blocks every day without symptoms.

Exam: BP: 120/70 mmHg, pulse: 90 bpm
Chest: Clear
Cardiac: Irregular rhythm, normal S_1 and S_2, no murmur
ECG: Atrial fibrillation with PVCs

Laboratory:
Hct: 38%
Glucose: 160 mg/dL

Which of the following would be the __most__ appropriate next step?

A. Proceed with surgery.
B. Obtain TTE before surgery.
C. Risk assess with dipyridamole thallium stress test.
D. Risk assess with cardiac catheterization.
E. Postpone surgery.

154.

You see a 24-year-old woman for a routine physical, when she begins to feel lightheaded and falls to the ground. She is unresponsive. No seizure activity is noted. Her vital signs are stable. Though she looks somewhat pale, she regains consciousness within 3 minutes and, within 15 minutes, is back to her previous state. She says that she felt weak, and the room became "dark" to her just prior to "falling out." She says that she has not been ill and otherwise has had no medical problems. She does admit to frequently feeling lightheaded upon rising quickly from the supine or seated positions, and says that she may have passed out once before in church.

Which of the following is the <u>most</u> likely explanation for her syncopal episode?

A. Hypertrophic cardiomyopathy
B. Anomalous coronary artery
C. Long QT syndrome
D. Severe aortic stenosis
E. Neurocardiogenic (vasovagal) syncope

155.

A 45-year-old man presents in cardiogenic shock. He is started on dopamine. His blood pressure rises nicely, and you begin a workup of his underlying cause.

Given that dopamine's results are dose-dependent, which dose is appropriate for this clinical condition?

A. < 2 μg/kg/min
B. 2–5 μg/kg/min
C. > 10 μg/kg/min
D. > 20 μg/kg/min

156.

A 25-year-old male presents after having a syncopal episode while playing basketball this morning. He has no other symptoms and says that he feels fine now.

Physical examination:
HEENT: Normal
Neck: Carotid pulse has a rapid upstroke and is bifid
Heart: RRR with a harsh, non-radiating midsystolic aortic murmur
Lungs: Normal
Abdomen: Benign
GU: Normal male genitalia
Skin: No rash

On further testing, he performs a Valsalva maneuver, and his murmur increases in intensity.

Which of the following is the <u>most</u> likely diagnosis?

    A. Coronary artery disease
    B. Abnormal coronary artery
    C. Mitral valve prolapse
    D. Aortic stenosis
    E. Hypertrophic cardiomyopathy

157.

A 40-year-old male comes into the emergency department for laceration repair after an altercation in a local bar.

As per routine, he is placed on a monitor and you note the following tracing:

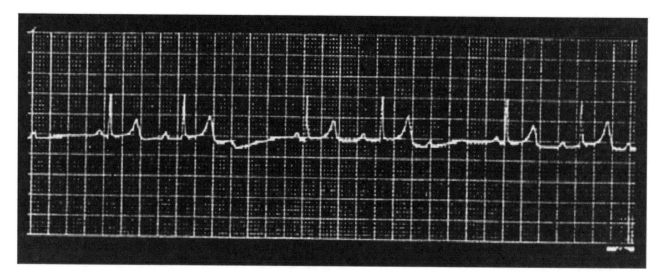

He has no other medical problems and is on no medications.

Which of the following would be the <u>most</u> appropriate next step?

    A. Temporary pacemaker
    B. Clinical electrophysiologic study
    C. Permanent pacemaker
    D. Observation only
    E. Begin an ACE inhibitor

158.

A 55-year-old man and his wife arrive at your hospital to visit a friend who is an inpatient. While waiting for an elevator, the man suddenly grabs his chest, hollers out in pain, and then falls against the back wall. A code is called and you respond. His wife reports that for 3 months, he has been having occasional episodes of pain in his chest that awakens him from sleep in the early morning. He never gets pain while doing chores at home, such as mowing the grass. He recently underwent an ECG and exercise stress test at his internist's office and was told his results were "normal." He is otherwise healthy. His only medicine is an aspirin a day that he self-prescribed at the onset of his chest pains. Family history is unremarkable. He does not smoke or use drugs.

Vital signs: HR: 120, respirations: 18, BP: 110/65 mmHg, afebrile
He is slightly confused. The physical exam is otherwise normal. There is no nuchal rigidity.
Within 15 minutes, he has regained normal mentation.
ECG during this episode: Sinus tachycardia with ST-segment depression in leads V1–V4.
ECG performed 15 minutes after recovery: Normal
Urgent echocardiogram shows normal LV wall motion with a normal estimated ejection fraction
Laboratory: cTn-I 30 minutes after the episode: < 0.01 ng/mL

Cardiac catheterization shows normal coronary arteries.

Which of the following is the <u>most</u> appropriate pharmacotherapy?

    A. Lidocaine
    B. Aspirin, propranolol, enalapril, and PRN nitrates
    C. Aspirin
    D. Aspirin, propranolol, enalapril, clopidogrel, and tirofiban
    E. Nitrates and calcium channel blockers

159.

A 56-year-old woman is admitted with an anterior MI. She was stabilized and initially received aspirin, thrombolytic therapy, heparin, nitrates, and beta-blockers. On day 4, she has multiple runs of ventricular tachycardia that are asymptomatic and last only a few seconds. Eventually, her thrombolytics and anticoagulants are discontinued. On day 6, she becomes acutely short of breath.

Vital signs: BP: 86/55 mmHg, pulse: 106 bpm, respiration: 19.
On exam, there is a systolic murmur that begins in mid-systole and extends to the second heart sound. It is audible over the entire chest.

Which of the following is the <u>most</u> appropriate next step in patient care?

    A. Take to the cath-lab and re-institute thrombolytic therapy for a recurrent MI.
    B. Immediately aspirate the pericardial sac for presumed tamponade.
    C. Prescribe massive volume resuscitation for presumed right ventricular infarction.
    D. Order an immediate surgical consultation for repair of a ruptured papillary muscle.
    E. Order an immediate surgical consultation for repair of a ventricular septal defect.

160.

A 59-year-old woman presents to the emergency department with acute shortness of breath and chest discomfort. She has a history of angina and intermittently takes nitroglycerin tablets when she has exertional chest pain.

Her ECG is presented here:

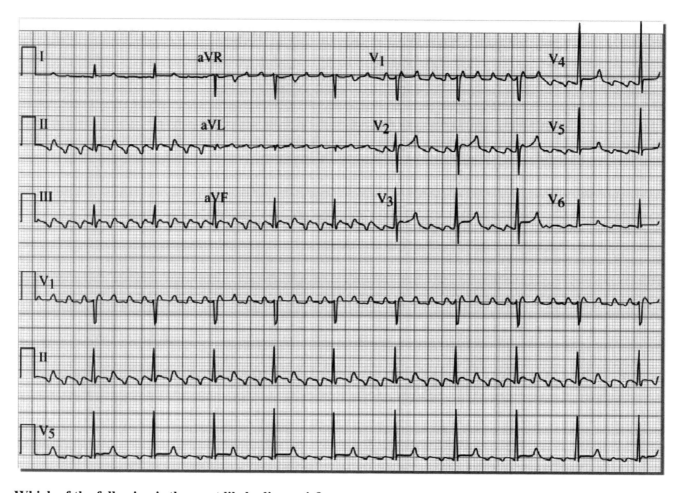

Which of the following is the <u>most</u> likely diagnosis?

    A. Sinus tachycardia
    B. Atrial fibrillation
    C. 2nd degree block, type 1
    D. Atrial flutter
    E. 3rd degree heart block

161.

A 52-year-old woman presents to the emergency department complaining of shortness of breath. Symptoms began acutely while the patient was mowing her backyard, but she continues to be short of breath even after rest. She denies chest pain, cough, orthopnea, paroxysmal nocturnal dyspnea, and lower extremity swelling or edema. For 3 months, she has experienced exertional fatigue and has had to rest while performing activities, such as grocery shopping or climbing a flight of stairs. Past medical history includes diabetes mellitus, hypothyroidism, and tobacco abuse (2 packs/day for 15 years). She takes metformin 1,000 mg bid, rosiglitazone 4 mg daily, and levothyroxine 100 mcg daily. Family history is significant for coronary artery disease and hyperlipidemia in her sister and father. She denies use of drugs or alcohol. Review of systems is significant for dizziness, weakness, and vague right upper quadrant pain, all of which began within the past 30 minutes, accompanying the shortness of breath.

Vital signs: BP: 96/52 mmHg, HR: 62, respirations: 26, afebrile
The physical exam is normal except for jugular venous distention and tender hepatomegaly, with a slow return of the hepatojugular reflux. Kussmaul sign is present. Pulmonary exam reveals normal vesicular breath sounds.

Laboratory results:
HbA1c: 10.2%
cTn-I @ initial: 1.30 ng/mL
cTn-I @ 30 minutes: 6.75 ng/mL

Electrocardiogram is as follows:

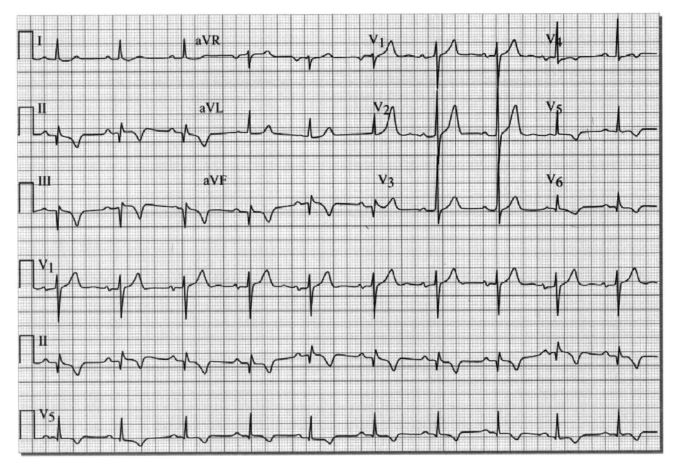

Which of the following is the <u>most</u> appropriate next step in patient care?

   A. Immediate angiography
   B. Aspirin plus intravenous nitroglycerin, labetalol, and enalapril
   C. Intravenous fluid resuscitation
   D. Intravenous nesiritide
   E. Intravenous dobutamine and furosemide

For this series of questions, we will go through the basic ECGs and rhythm strips that are "must knows" for the Board examination.

162.

Identify the following cardiac abnormality in lead II.

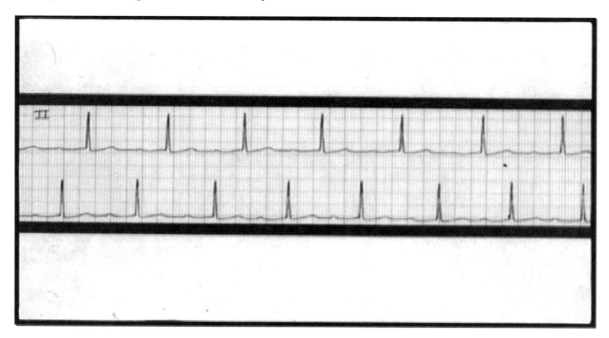

    A. Sinus tachycardia
    B. 1st degree AV block
    C. 2nd degree AV block, Mobitz 1
    D. 2nd degree AV block, Mobitz 2
    E. 3rd degree AV block

163.

Identify the following cardiac abnormality:

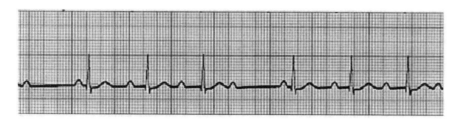

    A. Sinus tachycardia
    B. 1st degree AV block
    C. 2nd degree AV block, Mobitz 1
    D. 2nd degree AV block, Mobitz 2
    E. 3rd degree AV block

164.

Identify the following abnormality:

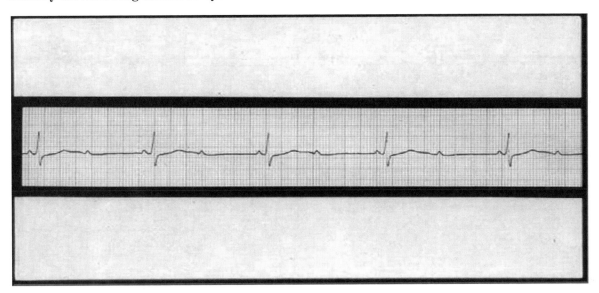

   A. Sinus tachycardia
   B. 1st degree AV block
   C. 2nd degree AV block, Mobitz 1
   D. 2nd degree AV block, Mobitz 2
   E. 3rd degree AV block

165.

Examine the following ECG and identify the abnormality:

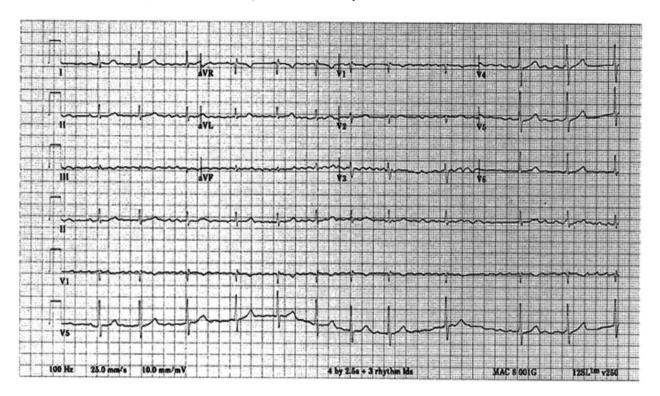

A. Ventricular tachycardia
B. Ventricular fibrillation
C. Atrial flutter
D. Atrial fibrillation
E. Normal sinus rhythm

166.

Review the following tracing and identify the appropriate rhythm:

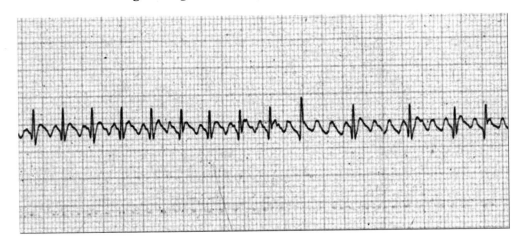

- A. Ventricular tachycardia
- B. Ventricular fibrillation
- C. Atrial flutter
- D. Atrial fibrillation
- E. Normal sinus rhythm

167.

Examine the following ECG and identify the abnormality:

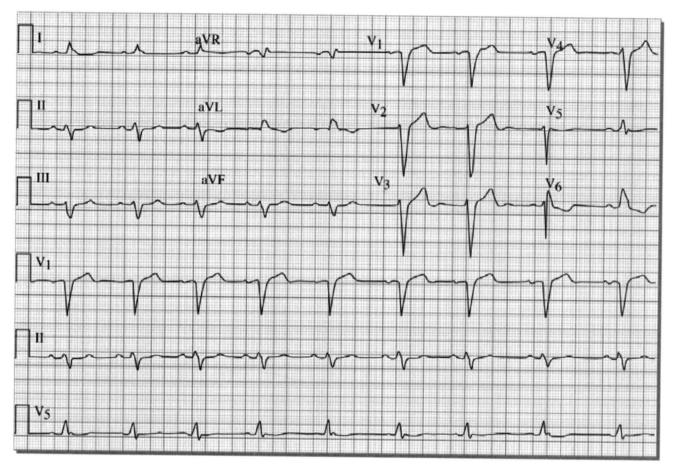

A. Ventricular tachycardia
B. Multifocal PVCs
C. Atrial fibrillation
D. Left bundle-branch block
E. Right bundle-branch block

168.

Examine the following ECG:

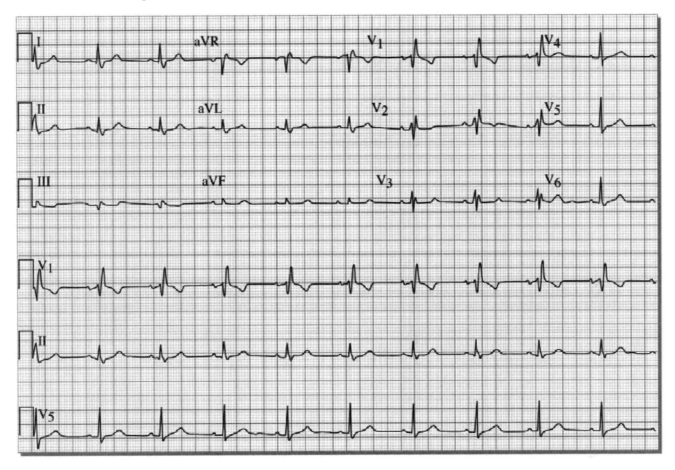

What is the underlying abnormality?

    A. Ventricular tachycardia
    B. Multifocal PVCs
    C. Atrial fibrillation
    D. Left bundle-branch block
    E. Right bundle-branch block

169.

The following patient had chest pain and positive enzymes for MI.

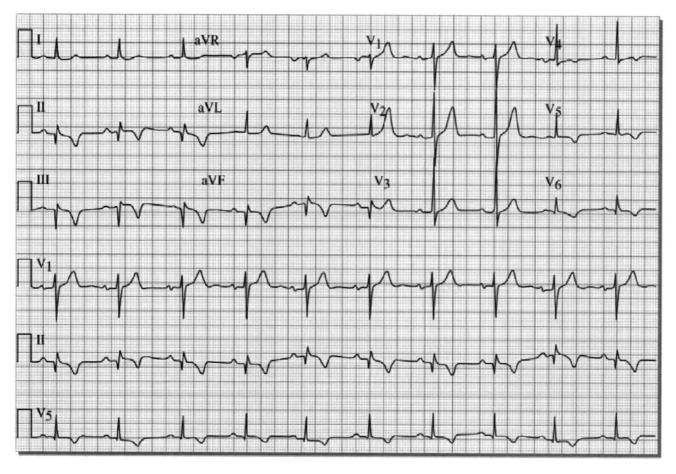

Where was the location of his MI based on the findings of his ECG?

    A. Transmural MI
    B. Anteroseptal
    C. Lateral MI
    D. Inferior MI
    E. Posterior MI

170.

Where does the ECG indicate that an MI has occurred?

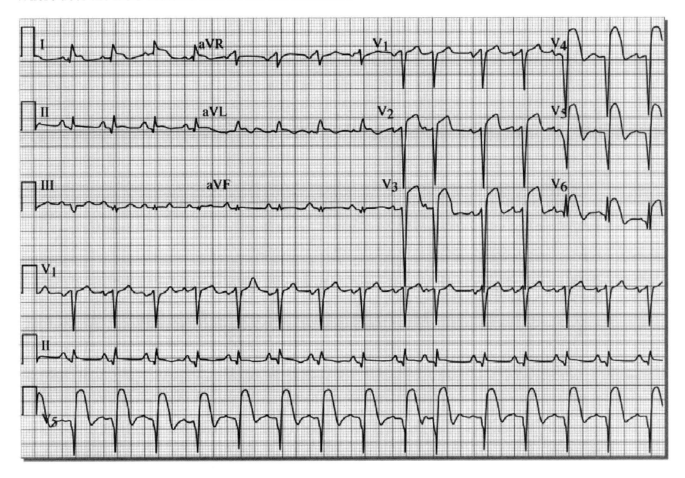

A. Lateral MI
B. Anterolateral MI
C. Posterior MI
D. Inferior MI
E. Septal MI

171.

What arrhythmia is this ECG demonstrating?

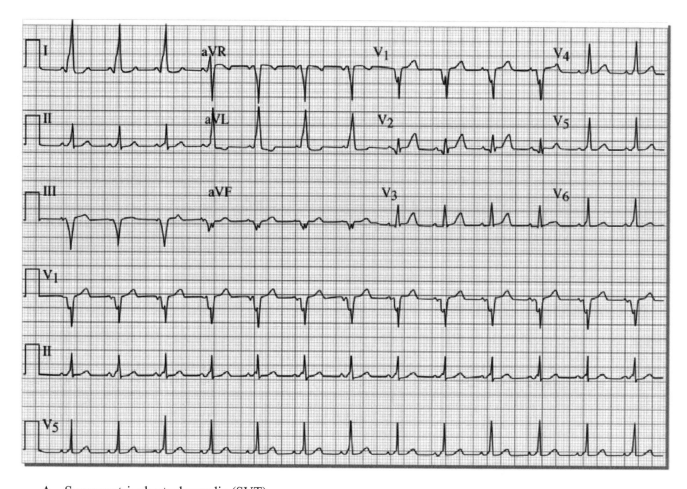

A. Supraventricular tachycardia (SVT)
B. Ventricular tachycardia
C. Atrial fibrillation
D. Wolff-Parkinson-White (WPW)
E. 2nd degree block, type 2

172.

Identify this ECG. For the most part, patients on the exam will present with chest discomfort and relief with leaning forward:

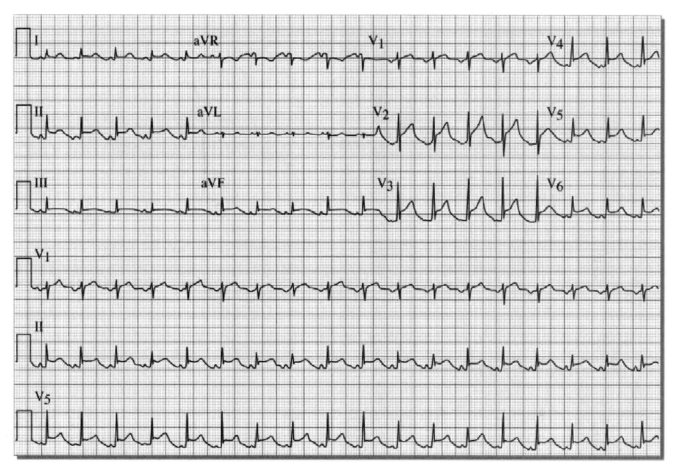

A. Acute anteroseptal MI
B. Posterior MI
C. Pericarditis
D. Digitalis toxicity
E. Wolff-Parkinson-White

173.

Know this next ECG!

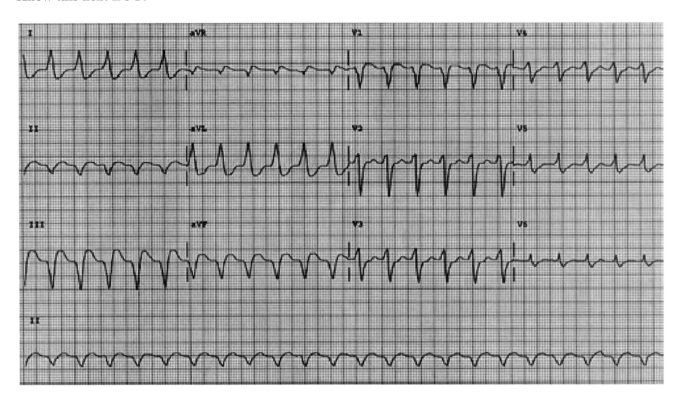

A. Atrial fibrillation
B. Atrial flutter
C. Ventricular fibrillation
D. Ventricular tachycardia
E. Supraventricular tachycardia

174.

A young patient has the following tracing on a routine ECG for a life insurance policy.

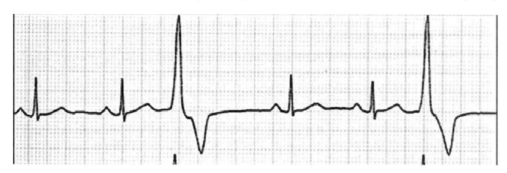

He is asymptomatic and denies symptoms. He has no abnormal physical findings.

What do you recommend?

  A. Overdrive pacing
  B. Beta-blocker therapy
  C. ACE inhibitor therapy
  D. Reassurance
  E. Treadmill stress test

INFECTIOUS DISEASE

175.

A 35-year-old woman with a history of bicuspid aortic valves presents with fever, extreme fatigue, anorexia, and malaise. Her temperature is 101.5° F. On physical examination, a previously noted systolic ejection click is associated with a new harsh ejection murmur. Additional clinical findings include mucous membrane and extremity petechiae and blanching, painless erythematous lesions on the palms and soles.

Which one of the following is the <u>most</u> likely cause of this patient's clinical signs and symptoms?

A. *Streptococcus pneumoniae*
B. Viridans streptococci
C. *Escherichia coli* O157:H7
D. *Neisseria meningitides*
E. *Haemophilus influenzae* type b

176.

A 50-year-old man presents for evaluation. He spent the night camping with a friend in a wooded community of rural New York state. During a shower following his return home, he discovered a brownish lump in the skin that he believed was a tick. He clearly states that the lump was not present in the morning when he was dressing. On physical examination, a tick is noted and removed from the left calf.

What is the best treatment option at this time?

A. Patient education and observation
B. Doxycycline for 14 days
C. Cephalexin for 14 days
D. Amoxicillin for 30 days
E. IV ceftriaxone for 7 days

177.

A 27-year-old man from North Carolina presents with a 48-hour history of fever, fatigue, anorexia, diffuse myalgias, and headache. Upon awakening on the day of presentation, he noticed a rash that continues to worsen. On physical examination, his temperature is 102.6° F. He appears ill and has an erythematous maculopapular and petechial rash that includes the trunk and, most prominently, the wrists, ankles, palms, and soles.

Which of the following laboratory findings is <u>most</u> likely to be identified in this patient?

A. Thrombocytosis
B. Elevated serum levels of amylase and lipase
C. Elevated WBC count associated with prominent lymphocytosis
D. Hyponatremia
E. Hyperkalemia

178.

A 48-year-old woman living in Arkansas presents complaining of a "swollen, infected and tender neck gland" associated with fever, nausea, and vomiting. On physical examination, her temperature is 103° F. Positive findings include a tender, fluctuant, and warm 2 x 1.5-cm anterior cervical lymph node and an ulcerative lesion with associated eschar formation located several inches below the node. Upon further questioning, she reports that she has recently been caring for a rabbit after it was bitten by their family dog.

Which of the following is the <u>most</u> appropriate choice of treatment for this patient?

    A. Cefotaxime
    B. Famciclovir
    C. Imipenem-cilastatin
    D. Gentamicin
    E. Itraconazole

179.

Following clinical evaluation for a febrile illness, a 25-year-old woman is thought to likely have an infection caused by adenovirus.

Which of the following findings is <u>most</u> likely to be associated with her illness?

    A. Inflammation of the bulbar and palpebral conjunctiva
    B. Enlargement of the spleen and liver
    C. Petechiae covering the extensor surfaces of the hands and feet
    D. Swelling of one or more large joints
    E. Ulcerative lesions covering the soft palate

180.

A 40-year-old woman from Connecticut presents with a history of subjective fever, myalgia, headache, and a rash, which she first noticed the day prior to presentation. On physical examination, her temperature is 100.6° F. A 3 x 5-cm circular erythematous lesion with central clearing is present on the left upper thigh. A similar but smaller lesion is located just below her left knee.

Which of the following complications often occurs later in the course of this illness in patients who do <u>not</u> initially receive appropriate treatment?

    A. Unilateral facial nerve palsy
    B. Symmetric proximal lower extremity weakness
    C. Miosis, ptosis, and anhidrosis
    D. Lower back pain associated with paresthesias in the lower extremity and urinary retention
    E. Temporary loss of vision associated with hemiparesis

181.

An 18-year-old woman is transported to the emergency room after being found lying on the street in a confused and disoriented state. Two friends accompany her and report that they and the patient have been "living on the streets." Upon arrival, she vomits and is incontinent of stool. On physical examination, she is lethargic but able to recognize her friends. Her temperature is 103.7° F and blood pressure is 88/40. A diffuse, generalized and intensely erythematous rash, associated with hyperemia of the conjunctiva and a "strawberry tongue," is noted in addition to 2 inflamed 4 x 6-cm superficial abrasions over her lower extremity. Laboratory results include elevated serum transaminases, a BUN of 55 mg/dL, and a serum creatinine of 2.7 mg/dL.

Which of the following is the <u>most</u> likely cause of this patient's symptoms?

    A. Viridans streptococci
    B. *Shigella flexneri*
    C. *Clostridium difficile*
    D. *Staphylococcus aureus*
    E. *Pseudomonas aeruginosa*

182.

A 30-year-old male immigrant, recently arriving from a remote area of the former Soviet Union, presents with a 2-day history of headache, generalized malaise, sore throat, and cough. His temperature is 101° F. Findings on physical examination include prominent suboccipital and postauricular lymphadenopathy and soft palate petechiae distributed among larger reddish spots.

Which of the following is the <u>most</u> likely cause of this patient's clinical signs and symptoms?

    A. Group A beta-hemolytic streptococcus
    B. Rubeola virus
    C. Rubella virus
    D. Coxsackievirus
    E. Epstein-Barr virus

183.

A 17-year-old girl presents with a 5–6-day history of malaise, headache, sore throat, and increased temperature. Findings on physical examination include periorbital and eyelid edema unassociated with changes in the conjunctiva, petechial lesions at the junction of the hard and soft palate, and an erythematous maculopapular morbilliform-like eruption on the trunk, upper arms, and thighs.

Which of the following is the <u>most</u> likely cause of her clinical signs and symptoms?

    A. Coxsackievirus A16
    B. Parvovirus B19
    C. Epstein-Barr virus
    D. Adenovirus
    E. Human herpesvirus 6

184.

A 26-year-old man presents with a 2-day history of pain in his proximal right arm associated with decreased range of motion and subjective fever. On physical examination, two 3 x 3.5-cm tender, slightly warm, right axillary lymph nodes are identified.

Which of the following additional findings is <u>most</u> likely to be identified if his clinical findings are the result of infection caused by *Bartonella henselae*?

    A. Several cutaneous papules
    B. Thickened yellowed nail plates
    C. Multiple small retinal hemorrhages associated with a whitish-pale center
    D. Nontender, small erythematous lesions on the palms or soles
    E. Painful erythematous raised lesions on the palms and soles

185.

You are asked to consult on a 26-year-old female who is 4 months pregnant and reported to the emergency department with concerns regarding meningitis exposure. The patient moved this week to your area to stay with her parents for the duration of her pregnancy. She was notified that her boyfriend, with whom she was in intimate contact with up to seven days ago, was hospitalized for meningococcal meningitis. Her family was contacted by the hospital recommending evaluation for his close contacts. The information conveyed indicated his cultures were (+) for *Neisseria meningitides* and was identified as serotype B.

Due to her contact history, which of the following is the <u>most</u> appropriate recommendation?

    A. Prescribe prophylactic rifampin therapy.
    B. Institute prophylactic ceftriaxone therapy.
    C. Recommend prophylactic ciprofloxacin therapy.
    D. Administer tetravalent polysaccharide meningococcal vaccine.
    E. Advise no treatment and close observation only.

186.

Physicians are required to report certain communicable diseases to appropriate public health agencies.

Which of the following conditions is designated as a notifiable disease on the national level in the United States?

    A. *Trichomonas*
    B. Syphilis
    C. *Gardnerella*
    D. Genital herpes
    E. Human papilloma virus

187.

A 45-year-old male is admitted through the emergency department with the diagnosis of community-acquired pneumonia. He presented with a three-day history of fever and chills associated with night sweats and generalized myalgias. He has developed productive cough and shortness of breath.

On physical examination, the patient is noted to have moderate tachypnea and scattered wheezes and rales on chest auscultation. His pulse oximeter on room air is 85%.

The chest radiograph is abnormal and reveals alveolar infiltrates with a reticulonodular pattern.

Blood and sputum cultures were obtained, and the patient was started on IV azithromycin with admission for observation.

As you are beginning rounds, you receive a call from pathology informing you that the sputum is most remarkable for a characteristic thick-walled yeast cell (8- to 15-mcg diameter) with broad-based daughter cells consistent with *Blastomyces dermatitidis*.

The most appropriate action at this time would be:

   A. Await culture confirmation of blastomycosis.
   B. Continue current antibiotic regimen.
   C. Change the antibiotic choice to itraconazole.
   D. Add ceftriaxone to the azithromycin coverage.
   E. Change the antibiotic choice to ketoconazole.

188.

A 52-year-old male presents to the local urgent care following an encounter with a neighborhood cat. The patient attempted to catch the cat that was frequently drinking from the family's fish pond and frightening the fish. He was scratched multiple times, and two or three bite marks seem to be present as well. The wounds are washed and irrigated extensively.

In considering prophylactic antibiotics for this person, which of the following would be the most appropriate choice?

   A. Erythromycin
   B. Clindamycin
   C. Cephalexin
   D. Dicloxacillin
   E. Amoxicillin-clavulanate

189.

A 25-year-old man presents for a routine physical exam. He has no chronic medical problems, takes no medications, and does not smoke or drink alcohol. He is gay, has been sexually active with one partner for the past 6 months, and reports sporadic condom use. He works as an accountant and has not traveled outside the U.S. His exam is normal. You suggest HIV testing, sexual risk counseling, and routine blood work for cholesterol. He has not had a recent PPD or CXR, and he has not had hepatitis A, hepatitis B, or pneumococcal vaccines.

Which of the following preventive health measures is also appropriate for him today?

A. Placing a PPD
B. Hepatitis A and B vaccines
C. Pneumococcal vaccine
D. Hepatitis A, hepatitis B, and pneumococcal vaccine
E. Screening chest radiograph

190.

A 54-year-old female with a long history of diabetes mellitus is admitted with cellulitis of her right foot. Three weeks ago, her podiatrist performed a surgical bunion removal, and on postoperative day 7, she developed erythema, drainage, and pain in the surgical site, which has worsened. She was admitted; the poorly healed wound was débrided, and deep tissue cultures were obtained. Radiographs obtained on postoperative day 21 did not reveal evidence of bone involvement, and blood cultures were negative. She was started on intravenous vancomycin and improved significantly. Cultures from the deep tissue grew *Staphylococcus aureus* with resistance to methicillin (MRSA) and sensitivity to clindamycin, trimethoprim/sulfamethoxazole, and levofloxacin.

The laboratory performed an erythromycin-clindamycin D-zone test, and the results are reported as positive. As the patient improves, arrangements are made for outpatient completion of antibiotic therapy.

Which of the following is the <u>most</u> appropriate outpatient antibiotic therapy?

A. Oral clindamycin
B. Oral amoxicillin-clavulanate
C. Oral trimethoprim/sulfamethoxazole
D. Oral vancomycin
E. Oral dicloxacillin

191.

A 19-year-old female presents to the emergency department with a one-day history of septic symptoms. She reports a significant toothache over the last three days; and, on the morning of presentation, she developed vomiting, diffuse muscle pain, fever, some confusion, and a diffuse erythematous, macular rash with nondescript borders. She has no medical history and is taking no medications. Her last menstrual cycle was 10 days previously and was normal.

On exam, she is in moderate distress. Her temperature is 38.9° C (102.0° F); heart rate is 136/min with weak peripheral pulses; blood pressure is 84/54 mmHg; and respiratory rate is 18/min. She has significant orthostatic changes. There is bilateral conjunctival erythema and significant swelling over the left maxillary area with an apparent complicated tooth abscess. There is significant hyperemia of the mucous membranes. Lungs demonstrate good air movement with clear auscultation. Cardiac exam reveals a rapid rate and no murmurs. Abdomen is unremarkable. Skin is erythematous and generally warm to the touch; no desquamation, blistering, or tenderness is noted.

Patient is started on aggressive intravenous hydration; blood and urine cultures are obtained; and she undergoes drainage of the dental abscess. She is also started on a broad-spectrum antibiotic.

Blood and urine cultures showed no growth, and cultures obtained during abscess drainage revealed Gram (+) cocci in clusters. *Staphylococcus aureus* grows in culture of the abscess.

Which of the following is the <u>most</u> likely explanation for these findings?

  A. Erysipelas
  B. Toxic shock syndrome
  C. Stevens-Johnson syndrome
  D. Staphylococcal scalded skin syndrome (SSSS)
  E. Toxic epidermal necrolysis

192.

You are called to evaluate an 83-year-old female resident of a long-term care facility with long-standing dementia. Nursing staff has noted increasing restlessness, generalized scratching, and a progressive rash. These symptoms have been progressing over the last 36 to 48 hours. The patient is unable to describe her complaints, but is persistently scratching and seems distressed. Exam reveals significant excoriations diffusely over the entire body, with greatest involvement at the wrists and waistbands of her underclothing. No significant crusting or cellulitis is noted. Her roommate, who was not under your care, was transferred five days ago to an inpatient setting after she developed extreme skin involvement with an extensive impetiginous rash.

On further examination of her hands, you notice what appear to be burrow-like structures:

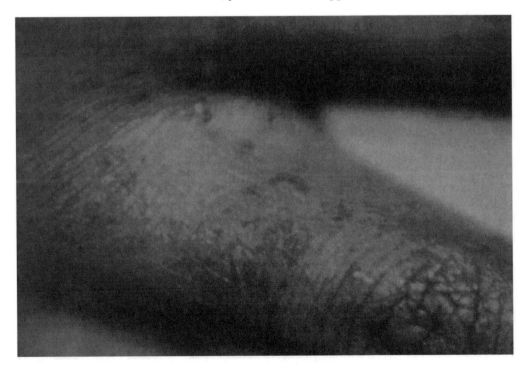

You do a scraping of one of the lesions and find this:

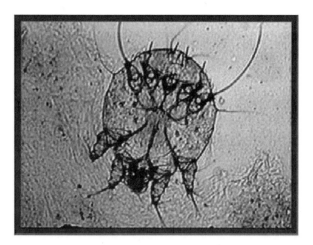

Which of the following is the <u>most</u> appropriate therapy?

A. Oral ampicillin-sulbactam
B. Oral diphenhydramine
C. Topical calamine
D. Topical permethrin
E. Topical steroids

193.

You are consulted to evaluate a 28-year-old Hispanic patient in the ICU after a motor vehicle accident. He was thrown from a car and sustained extensive trauma to the skin of his back, legs, and right upper extremity. His family recently immigrated to the area from Central America. Local family members were involved in the accident and are unable to provide medical information. His previous immunization status is unknown. The trauma surgeons have asked your advice regarding recommendations for tetanus prophylaxis.

Which of the following immunizations should be administered at this time?

A. Diphtheria, tetanus toxoid and acellular pertussis (DTaP) vaccine and tetanus immune globulin (TIG)
B. Tdap vaccine alone
C. Tdap in combination with tetanus immune globulin (TIG)
D. TIG with follow-up Tdap tetanus vaccine in six weeks

194.

You are asked to evaluate an 85-year-old female resident of an extended care facility who suffers from marked dementia. Nursing staff reports two nights of marked irritability, poor sleep, and complaints of rectal irritation. She has had no fever, diarrhea, or reported trauma. The patient is alert and is in no apparent distress at the time of examination. Her vitals are within normal limits. The rectal exam is remarkable for significant perirectal irritation with mild erythema and excoriations with thickening of the perirectal skin. The involvement of the skin is limited to the gluteal fold region and is not painful to palpation. No palpable masses or "discharge" is noted. No fissures are noted, and the external vaginal area is unremarkable.

A "scotch tape" test is done and shows the following:

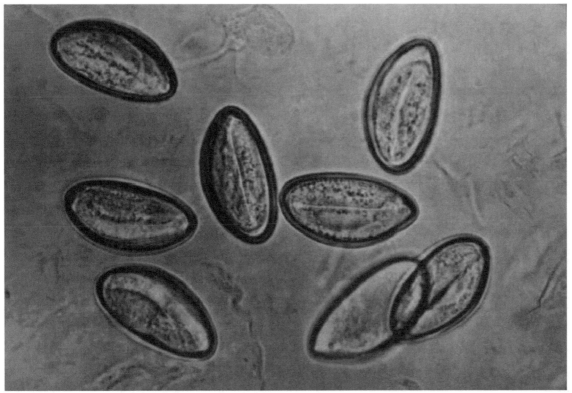

Which of the following is the <u>most</u> appropriate pharmacotherapy?

A. Oral albendazole
B. Topical nystatin
C. Oral cephalexin
D. Topical hydrocortisone
E. Topical permethrin

195.

You are called to see a 64-year-old female patient admitted during the evening with abdominal pain, fever, and a working diagnosis of diverticulitis. Patient was started on IV fluids and antibiotics. During the night, however, she developed erythematous induration of the skin over the left lower abdomen; the area is now becoming violaceous with blister formation and has extended toward the left flank and left hypochondrial region. She is complaining of significant pain and rigors. You direct the nurse to obtain immediate blood cultures and order appropriate pain medications.

Which of the following is the <u>most</u> appropriate next step in management to prevent morbidity?

A. Emergent surgical exploration and debridement
B. Immediate change of antibiotics to clindamycin, ampicillin-sulbactam, and gentamicin
C. Leading-edge aspiration or tissue biopsy for Gram stain and culture
D. STAT contrast tomography of the abdomen

196.

You are asked to evaluate a 27-year-old otherwise healthy man whose dog bit him yesterday. The animal has not been ill and receives regular veterinary check-ups and vaccinations. The patient has no symptoms, no fevers, and is otherwise healthy. His last tetanus booster was 7 years ago.

On exam, he appears well and is afebrile. His left second finger is swollen and erythematous, and he has pain with grasp. He reports numbness over the distal and mid-finger. There is no lymphadenopathy, and no erythema is noted on the arm.

Which of the following is the <u>most</u> appropriate intervention?

    A. Immediate incision and drainage, parenteral antibiotics, no Tdap booster, no rabies vaccine
    B. Tdap booster, oral amoxicillin-clavulanate, observation, no rabies vaccine
    C. No Tdap booster, oral amoxicillin-clavulanate, observation, no rabies vaccine
    D. Tdap booster, IV ampicillin-sulbactam, begin rabies vaccine, consultation with hand surgeon
    E. Tdap booster, IV ampicillin-sulbactam, no rabies vaccine, consultation with hand surgeon

197.

Your patient is a 32-year-old male brought to the emergency department from the county jail for an infected hand. He was involved in a bar fight 4 days previously, in which he received multiple wounds to his right hand after striking another bar patron several times in the mouth. The victim of the assault fled before police arrived, and his identity is unknown. The patient has an extensive history of alcohol use. Review of records from previous hospital visits indicates that the patient has a significant allergy to penicillin. He received a documented tetanus booster 4 years previously. No other vaccine history is available.

The patient has several open, draining wounds across the dorsal aspect of the fingers and right hand. Each is surrounded by significant erythema. X-ray of his hand does not demonstrate any fractures or foreign body.

After debridement of necrotic tissue and cleaning of the wound sites by an experienced hand surgeon, which of the following is the <u>most</u> appropriate intervention?

    A. Institution of trimethoprim/sulfamethoxazole only
    B. Administration of hepatitis B vaccine
    C. Closure of the wounds to promote healing
    D. Administration of tetanus toxoid–diphtheria-acellular pertussis (Tdap) booster
    E. Administration of hepatitis B immune globulin (HBIG) and hepatitis B vaccine

198.

You are about to discharge a 62-year-old man from the hospital after a GI bleed, which was determined to be caused by an AV malformation in the colon. He feels well and has no symptoms. His past medical history consists of mild, diet-controlled hyperlipidemia and cataracts. He is a life-long nonsmoker.

He was initially admitted to the MICU with anemia, but was stepped down after 24 hours and has had an uncomplicated hospital course since then. It is now hospital day #3, and his hemoglobin remains stable at 10. He has had an indwelling Foley catheter and a peripheral central venous catheter since admission to the MICU.

On exam, he is afebrile, and the exam is normal.

WBC: 7,600 cells/mm^3
Urinalysis performed on day #2: 3+ bacteria, 10 WBC/hpf, 0 RBC/hpf, nitrite-negative
Urine culture: *E. coli* > 10^5 cfu/mL; sensitive to ampicillin

Which of the following is the <u>most</u> appropriate management?

    A. No antibiotics, remove Foley and peripheral central venous catheters, discharge to home.
    B. Oral antibiotics, remove Foley and peripheral central venous catheters, discharge to home.
    C. IV antibiotics, remove Foley catheter, delay discharge 24 hours, repeat U/A and culture.
    D. Oral antibiotics, remove Foley and peripheral central venous catheters, delay discharge, repeat U/A in 24 hours, discharge without antibiotics if U/A is negative.

199.

A 21-year-old man is evaluated for a rash and fever. He states he has felt sick for the past 3 weeks with "flu-like" symptoms that progressed to fever, fatigue, and muscle aches. He took some left-over amoxicillin from an episode of pharyngitis 6 months ago, and subsequently developed a reddish rash over his trunk and extremities.

The rash on his left arm is shown here:

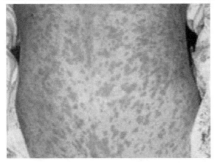

He takes no other medications and has no risks for HIV infection. He is up-to-date with immunizations. He does not smoke cigarettes, uses alcohol only on weekends, and does not use "recreational" drugs. Physical exam shows an ill-appearing but well-nourished young man. Temperature is 38.8° C (101.8° F); otherwise vital signs are normal. There are multiple tender anterior and posterior cervical lymph nodes. There is a pharyngeal exudate, and you note a few petechiae on the palate. A "fullness" is palpable in the left upper quadrant. He has an erythematous, morbilliform rash on his chest, back, arms, and legs.

Which of the following is the <u>most</u> appropriate next step in management to prevent morbidity?

    A. Counsel the patient to abstain from alcohol.
    B. Counsel the patient to abstain from sulfa-based antibiotics.
    C. Counsel the patient to abstain from estuarine water exposure.
    D. Counsel the patient to abstain from contact sports.
    E. Counsel the patient to abstain from sun exposure.

200.

A 32-year-old Peace Corps volunteer presents to your office 3 weeks after returning from central Africa, complaining of fever, malaise, headache, and mild diarrhea. He spent his last 3 months providing medical care to a small village. He has no previous medical illnesses. He does not drink alcohol and smokes half a pack of cigarettes per day. He received yellow fever and hepatitis A vaccines before the trip. He was given mefloquine for the trip to Africa, which he took weekly during his stay there. He is currently taking only acetaminophen, as needed for the fever and headache. He denies having any sexual contacts during his stay in Africa.

On physical exam, he appears ill and fatigued. His blood pressure is 112/70 mmHg, pulse 88 bpm, respirations 14/min, and temperature 102.4° F (39.1° C).

There is no jaundice, but scleral icterus is present. ENT exam is normal. There is no lymphadenopathy. Heart is regular with no murmur; lungs are clear; and abdominal exam is normal with no hepatosplenomegaly. There is no peripheral edema. He is lethargic, but his neurologic exam is nonfocal. There is no rash.

Laboratory results:

WBC:	10.7 cells/mm^3
Hgb:	12.2 mg/dL
Hct:	37%
Platelets:	81,000 cells/mm^3
Glucose:	92 mg/dL
BUN:	30 mg/dL
Creatinine:	1.2 mg/dL
AST:	20 U/L
ALT:	22 U/L
Alk Phos:	100 U/L
Total Bili:	3.6 mg/dL
Direct Bili:	0.9 mg/dL

Several peripheral smears are done and show ring-shaped organisms within erythrocytes, with some of the RBCs infected with multiple organisms. One of the peripheral smears shows the following:

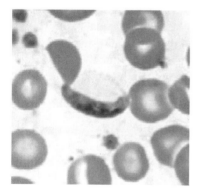

Which of the following is the <u>most</u> appropriate initial step in patient care?

    A. High-dose chloroquine alone
    B. Chloroquine followed by two weeks of primaquine
    C. Artemether-lumefantrine
    D. Doxycycline alone
    E. Exchange transfusion

201.

The daughter of a divorced 36-year-old woman brings her to your office because she has been "acting strange" for the past week. The family has noted that she has been sleeping less, is "always jittery," has begun to forget things (recent events, names); and today, she placed her boots in the refrigerator. She has no history of chronic medical disease or mental illness. She takes no medications, does not smoke cigarettes, drinks a glass of wine 3–4 times a week, and has never done illicit drugs. She has had 6 sexual partners in the past two years.

ROS is significant only for subjective fevers for the past few days.

On physical exam, vital signs are normal, and the exam is nonfocal with the exception of the neurologic exam. The patient appears manic; mini-mental status exam score is 24/30. Cranial nerves are intact. Motor and sensory exam are normal. Gait is slightly ataxic; she is unwilling to perform finger-to-nose testing. Reflexes are 2+ and symmetric.

Basic laboratory testing is unremarkable, including complete blood counts and metabolic panel.

MRI of the brain is performed. There is abnormal signal intensity in the left temporal lobe with slight mass effect.

Which of the following is the <u>most</u> likely diagnosis?

  A. HSV encephalitis
  B. Temporal lobe epilepsy
  C. Brain abscess
  D. Glioblastoma multiforme
  E. Schizoaffective disorder

202.

A 28-year-old female in her third month of pregnancy is referred to you by her obstetrician for recommendations regarding malaria prophylaxis. The patient is anticipating a 6-week church mission trip to a chloroquine-resistant malarial area. Despite recommendations to defer the trip, the patient is adamant on completing her travel plans.

Which of the following is the <u>most</u> appropriate anti-malarial pharmacotherapy?

  A. Mefloquine
  B. Atovaquone-proguanil
  C. Doxycycline
  D. Frequent applications of topical 70% DEET

203.

Conjugated meningococcal vaccine (Menactra®, Menveo®) is recommended for all adolescents today but particularly for military recruits, college students living in dormitories, and travelers to endemic areas of meningococcal disease.

Vaccination with conjugated meningococcal vaccine is also specifically recommended for patients with which of the following diseases?

A. Chronic asthma
B. Sickle cell disease
C. Cystic fibrosis
D. Epilepsy

204.

You are scheduled to see a 54-year-old female in your clinic as an emergency department follow-up. The patient was seen for a painful, vesicular rash in a dermatomal distribution on her left chest that developed over a 6-hour period. The emergency department physician made a diagnosis of shingles and started valacyclovir. She does give a past history of chicken pox as a child.

The patient is currently not working outside of the home, but regularly provides supervision of her grandchildren while their parents are at work.

Which of the following is the <u>most</u> appropriate recommendation?

A. Counsel that she should avoid contact with children infected with varicella zoster during the infectious phase to reduce the risk of developing zoster.
B. Counsel that primary infection with varicella zoster in adults usually restricts itself to a single dermatomal presentation.
C. Counsel that a single dose of varicella vaccine is adequate for susceptible adults to induce immunity to a zoster infection.
D. Counsel that valacyclovir or famciclovir started in the first 48 hours of a zoster flare can reduce the duration of post-herpetic neuralgia.

205.

An 18-year-old male patient presents to your office complaining of rash and watery diarrhea for the last 10 days. He has no significant past medical history and no history of allergies. He denies fevers or muscle ache, but does note some occasional, diffuse abdominal pain and "achy joints" that have been bothering him more for the last 2 days. He recently returned from a visit to North Carolina with his grandfather. There they hiked several days in the Great Smoky Mountains. On exam, the patient is febrile with temperature of 100° F (37.7° C). He denies pruritus.

The following rash is noted:

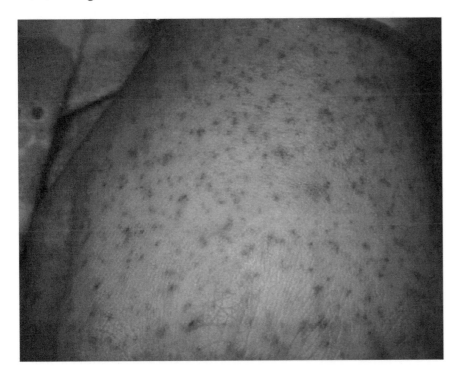

Which of the following is the <u>most</u> appropriate next step in patient care?

A. Send blood for serology and start erythromycin.
B. Perform immunofluorescent staining on a biopsy of the petechial lesions and then have the patient return in three days for follow-up of the results.
C. Start doxycycline and send blood for serology.
D. Start ceftriaxone 2 grams IV q 24 hours and send blood for serology.

206.

A 40-year-old man presents with a chief complaint of swelling in his groin for about a week. He lives in Missouri and is an avid hunter and fisherman. He says that he was out hunting raccoons 3 weeks ago and slept with his dog under an old oak tree. He is unsure if he received any tick bites. His appetite is depressed compared to normal, and he has had fever to 102° F (38.9° C) with some chills.

On physical examination, you note that he is 5'10" and weighs 280 lbs. The examination is otherwise significant only for a large right inguinal lymph node with a large eschar just proximal to the node (see picture that follows):

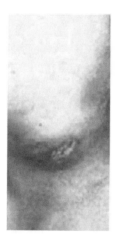

What is the <u>most</u> likely etiology for this illness?

    A. *Yersinia pestis*
    B. Leptospires
    C. *Francisella tularensis*
    D. *Ehrlichia chaffeensis*
    E. *Bordetella pertussis*

207.

A 20-year-old woman presents to the emergency department with septic shock. She was found by her boyfriend this morning sprawled on the kitchen floor and unresponsive. He reports she was well yesterday. You note that her skin appears red. She has fever and hypotension. Her boyfriend noted that she began having diarrhea last night and that she had started her menses yesterday. Laboratory results reveal pancytopenia, markedly elevated liver enzymes, and a creatinine of 2.3 mg/dL.

Which microorganism is <u>most</u> likely responsible for her acute presentation?

    A. *E. coli* O157:H7
    B. *Staphylococcus aureus*
    C. *Streptococcus pneumoniae*
    D. *Neisseria meningitidis*
    E. *Streptococcus agalactiae*

208.

An 80-year-old woman comes to your office with a 5-day history of fever, severe diarrhea, and increased urinary frequency. She develops hypotension, end-organ failure, and requires admission to the intensive care unit. The woman lives with her daughter and her family. They own a dog, cat, ferret, and turtle, but the patient has not had direct contact with the ferret or turtle. The daughter mentions that the turtle bowl is cleaned in the family kitchen sink. Cultures of her urine, stool, and blood all yield the same organism.

The patient's cultures will <u>most</u> likely grow which of the following organisms?

A. *Shigella*
B. *Salmonella*
C. *Pasteurella*
D. *Carmenella*
E. *E. coli* O157:H7

209.

A 33-year-old woman returns from a visit to central Africa. She reports good adherence to her malarial prophylaxis during her trip. She continues to take her mefloquine as directed on returning home. You receive a notification from the CDC that travelers to the country she visited are at risk for a type of malaria that has hypnozoite forms, and that primaquine must be taken as well on return to the United States.

Which species of malaria require the use of adjunctive primaquine to prevent the relapsing form of malaria?

A. *P. ovale* and *P. falciparum*
B. *P. ovale* and *P. vivax*
C. *P. ovale, P. vivax,* and *P. malariae*
D. *P. vivax* and *P. malariae*
E. *P. falciparum* only

210.

A 32-year-old, otherwise healthy man is brought by ambulance to the emergency department for confusion and hypoxia. His wife called EMS after returning from work and found him febrile and confused, lying in the bed. During the morning, he reported feeling unwell and decided not to go to work, but he was not confused and looked well. At lunch, when his wife called, he was also fairly well but reported having developed a fever. He has no medical history and takes no medications. For the past 3 days, he had been keeping a bedside vigil for his brother who accompanied him on the hunting trip and succumbed to a case of "severe pneumonia" yesterday.

He works as a postal worker in New Mexico, and his wife reports that he handles "suspicious packages all the time." He is an avid hunter and returned 4 days ago from a 7-day deer hunt in northern New Mexico, where they stayed in a cabin. He and his brother both killed a deer; his wife does not know whether he wears gloves while field dressing the animals. She reports he sustained several tick bites, and several rodents were noted in the cabin. He does not smoke or use drugs.

Physical examination: T 103.8° F, HR 125, RR 32, BP 95/60, Pulse oximetry on room air: 85%

He is cyanotic, confused, and somnolent.

Nuchal rigidity is absent. Head and neck examination is normal.

He is tachypneic with shallow respirations and coughing profusely with blood-tinged sputum. Coarse crackles are audible throughout.

Heart rate is tachycardic but regular.

Abdomen and skin exam is normal.

He moves all his extremities; cranial nerves appear normal.

Chest radiograph reveals diffuse, bilateral consolidations.

Assuming the patient acquired his infection from his brother, which of the following is the <u>most</u> likely pathogen?

    A. *Bacillus anthrax*
    B. *Francisella tularensis*
    C. *Yersinia pestis*
    D. *Clostridium botulinum*
    E. *Salmonella typhi*

211.

A 26-year-old man presents to the emergency department with fever and new-onset seizures. He has been acting erratically; and this morning, he thought he was the King of Nigeria. Prior to arrival, he had 2 episodes of tonic-clonic seizures, and upon arrival to the emergency department, he seized a third time. He was given lorazepam and a loading dose of phenytoin.

On physical examination, he appears agitated and confused.

Temperature 100.3° F (37.9° C), BP 120/65 mmHg, P 120 bpm, and oxygen saturation 97% on room air.

Blood glucose level at bedside = 98 mg/dL.

HEENT:	PERRLA, EOMI
	No papilledema
	No lacerations or bruising
Neck:	No meningismus
Heart:	Regular rate without murmurs, rubs, or gallops
Lungs:	Symmetric excursions, resonant to percussion, vesicular breath sounds throughout
Abdomen:	Normal bowel sounds, no hepatosplenomegaly
Extremities:	No cyanosis, clubbing, or edema
Neuro:	Sedated and unable to follow commands
	No gross facial asymmetry noted
	Gag reflex intact
	Appropriate responses to noxious stimuli
	Well-developed musculature
	No rigidity noted
	Reflexes were equal and symmetrical bilaterally

Initial Laboratory:

WBC:	12,000/μL
Hgb:	13.0 g/dL
Plt:	404,000/μL
Sodium:	134 mEq/L
Potassium:	3.7 mEq/L

Chloride:	92 mEq/L
Carbon dioxide:	26 mmol/L
BUN:	10 mg/dL
Creatinine:	1.1 mg/dL
Drug screen:	Negative
CXR:	Normal
CT of Brain:	No mass lesions; no hemorrhages.
LP:	Opening pressure: 18 cm H_2O
	176 WBC/µL (90% lymphocytes)
	760 RBC/µL
	70 mg/dL glucose
	95 mg/dL protein
	Gram stain, acid-fast smear, and cryptococcal antigen negative.
Serum RPR:	Negative

Which of the following tests is the <u>most</u> sensitive for discerning HSV as a cause of meningoencephalitis?

    A. MRI of the head
    B. EEG
    C. CT of the head
    D. Virus culture of cerebrospinal fluid (CSF)
    E. Polymerase chain reaction (PCR) testing of CSF

212.

A 30-year-old man was running through the cornfields near his home when he sustained a puncture wound from a nail that pierced his tennis shoe. Six days later, his foot is swollen, and he develops fever. A bone scan confirms osteomyelitis.

Which of the following is the <u>most</u> appropriate empiric pharmacotherapy?

    A. Nafcillin
    B. Ceftriaxone
    C. Trimethoprim/sulfamethoxazole
    D. Ciprofloxacin
    E. Tetracycline

213.

A healthy 25-year-old woman works as a lifeguard at the local swimming pool. She comes to your office because of redness and tearing of her right eye. She denies pain, saying she is experiencing only slight discomfort. She says that there are several kids and adults at the pool with obvious red eyes. She also says it is hard for her to differentiate whether their eyes are red "from chlorine or from diseases."

Review of systems is negative for diarrhea, abdominal pain, skin rashes, and fever blisters.

On exam, her right eye demonstrates conjunctival injection without obvious ulceration. There is increased lacrimation. Pupillary response and extraocular movements are normal.

Fluorescein stain of her eye reveals no abnormalities.

Here is a picture of her eye:

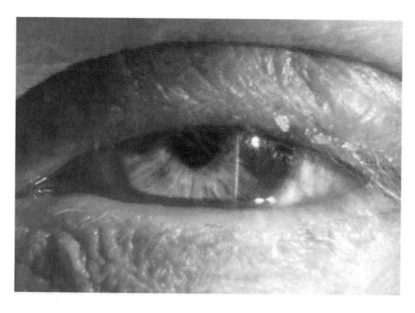

Which of the following is the _most_ likely pathogen?

A. *Mycobacterium tuberculosis*
B. *Mycobacterium marinum*
C. Adenovirus
D. *Histoplasma capsulatum*
E. *Vibrio vulnificus*

214.

A 50-year-old woman from Texas reports having experienced several tick bites in the last 3–4 years while camping in the Texas Panhandle. She presents with complaints of "chronic fatigue" and believes she has Lyme disease. She denies a rash or arthritis, and she has never been hospitalized for meningitis or carditis. Her only complaint is the fatigue, and she requests that you perform testing for Lyme disease.

Which of the following is the _most_ appropriate next step in diagnosis?

A. *B. burgdorferi* IgG.
B. *B. burgdorferi* IgM and IgG.
C. PCR for *B. burgdorferi*.
D. *B. burgdorferi* IgM, IgG, and PCR.
E. No additional testing is recommended.

215.

A 38-year-old man presents to the emergency department complaining of a rash, fever, and swelling of his left 2nd and 3rd metacarpal joints for the past two days. He states that while visiting his sister several weeks ago, he noticed a red rash on the cheeks of his niece, age 6. The child was otherwise well. Review of systems is negative for abdominal pain, bloody diarrhea, recent new sexual contacts, malar rash, and photosensitivity. The rash is described as "lacy" and constantly present, regardless of temperature.

On examination, he is febrile to 102° F (38.8° C), HR 126.
Physical exam is normal except for active synovitis of the 2nd and 3rd MCP joints on the left hand.

A diffuse, slightly erythematous reticular rash is present on his trunk, abdomen, and extremities.

There is no lymphadenopathy or hepatosplenomegaly.

CBC is normal.

Ferritin 250 ng/mL (normal 12–150 ng/mL)

His rash and the swelling of his fingers are noted below:

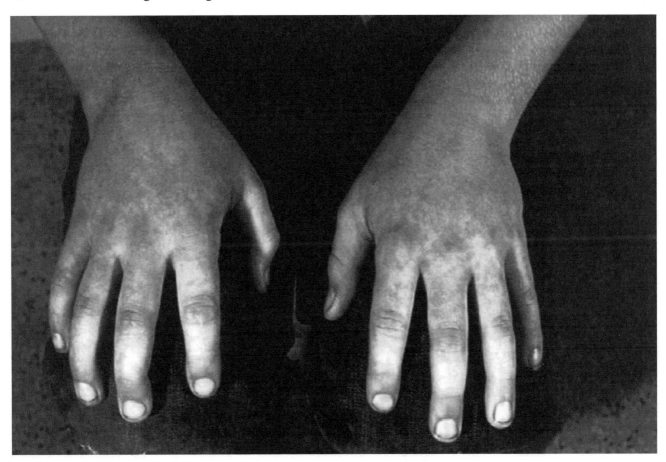

Which of the following is the _most_ likely diagnosis?

A. Rheumatoid arthritis
B. Coxsackievirus
C. Parvovirus B19
D. Still's disease
E. Echovirus

216.

A 60-year-old nurse presents with new onset of fever and chills. 10 days ago, she developed flu-like symptoms of fever, runny nose, cough, and severe myalgias. An influenza test was performed and was positive. The fever lasted seven days then remitted, and she began improving. However, over the past 24 hours, she has developed a new cough with left-sided pleuritic chest pain.

She appears in mild distress.

Chest radiograph reveals LLL consolidation.

Blood cultures grow the following organism:

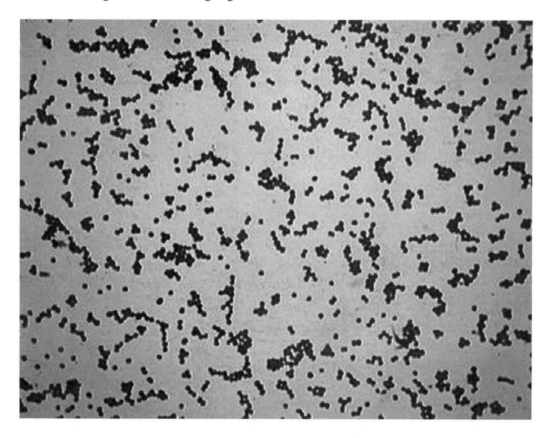

What is the most appropriate pharmacotherapy?

A. Oral amoxicillin-clavulanic acid (Augmentin®)
B. Vancomycin
C. Ceftriaxone
D. IV trimethoprim/sulfamethoxazole
E. Piperacillin-tazobactam

217.

While taking out her garbage to the curb, a 35-year-old woman steps on a rusty old can and punctures her foot. As she hobbled back to her house, she stepped in dog feces.

She reports having had all her childhood immunizations and a Tdap booster 4 years ago.

Which of the following immunizations should be administered at this time?

A. Td only
B. DTaP only
C. Td and Tetanus IG
D. DTaP and Tetanus IG
E. No further immunization at this time

218.

You see a 46-year-old female in the emergency department with initial complaints of blurred vision, followed by difficulty with swallowing, and increasing difficulty breathing. The symptoms began several hours after a family gathering where traditional foods were consumed. Communication with family indicates that several other members are also experiencing symptoms but with fewer difficulties.

The patient deteriorates and requires intubation and ventilatory support. Over the next several hours, other family members also present with worsening and similar symptoms.

A child, who was at the family gathering, presents with the following flaccid paralysis:

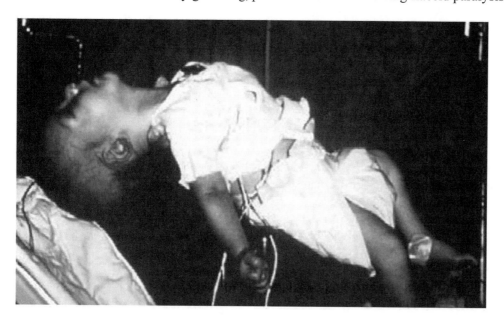

Which of the following is the <u>most</u> likely offending agent?

A. *Bacillus cereus*
B. *Clostridium botulinum*
C. Enterotoxigenic *E. coli*
D. *Shigella*

219.

A 25-year-old male presents with acute arthritis of his left knee. He has a history of recurrent sore throats over the past year. Sometimes he went to the physician, and other times he ignored the symptoms, and the soreness improved. He has had persistent fever with the onset of the arthritis. When you listen to his heart, you hear a new systolic murmur that was not there 2 years ago. A throat culture for group A streptococcus is negative.

Which of the following do you tell this patient about rheumatic fever?

A. Group A streptococcal skin infections can be responsible for rheumatic fever.
B. Diagnosis of acute rheumatic fever in an adult presenting with migratory arthritis and a new heart murmur requires confirmatory evidence of recent group A streptococcal infection.
C. Prophylactic antibiotic therapy is not necessary for those with rheumatic fever who do not have carditis.
D. Acute rheumatic fever usually occurs within the first week of untreated group A streptococcus infection.

220.

A 25-year-old nursing student works on an AIDS ward in New Jersey. While emptying out the urine bag from an HIV-infected patient (viral load > 500,000 copies/cc), some of the urine splashed onto her ungloved hand. No lesions were noted on her hand, and she does not have any noticeable breaks in the skin. She immediately washed her hand with soap and water and poured bleach over the area. The urine was light yellow in color.

She presents to the emergency room for follow-up care approximately 2 hours after the splash.

Which of the following should be recommended to prevent morbidity?

    A. Perform a genotype on the infected patient and initiate therapy based on results of the genotype (i.e., to determine if the patient has resistant virus).
    B. Start AZT + 3TC (Combivir®) only.
    C. Start 3-drug therapy.
    D. Start zidovudine only.
    E. No treatment is recommended.

221.

A 24-year-old otherwise healthy day care worker presents with signs and symptoms of meningitis that developed 10 days after a cold. Lumbar puncture (LP) is performed.

LP results:
Opening pressure: 210 cm H_2O
WBC: 4000/μL with 85% granulocytes
RBC: 20/μL
Total protein: 300 mg/dL
Glucose: 10 mg/dL (serum is 98 mg/dL)

It is 3 a.m. and the Gram stain cannot be completed until the morning laboratory crew arrives.

Which of the following is the <u>most</u> appropriate empiric pharmacotherapy?

    A. IV ampicillin and IV gentamicin
    B. IV ceftriaxone
    C. IV vancomycin
    D. IV vancomycin and IV ceftriaxone
    E. IV vancomycin and IV gentamicin

222.

A 70-year-old man presents to your office with symptoms of epididymitis. He denies sexual activity, especially since his sildenafil citrate prescription ran out 6 months ago. He is monogamous and has never had a sexually transmitted disease.

Which of the following is the <u>most</u> likely pathogen?

    A. *Chlamydia trachomatis.*
    B. *Neisseria gonorrhoeae.*
    C. *E. coli.*
    D. *Chlamydia trachomatis* or *Neisseria gonorrhoeae* is equally likely.
    E. *Pseudomonas aeruginosa.*

223.

A 70-year-old man presents with a painless lesion on his penis. He says that he had his sildenafil citrate prescription refilled 2 months ago and had unprotected sex with a prostitute 4 weeks ago while visiting Orlando. His rapid plasma reagin (RPR) and MHA-TP are positive.

A picture of the penile lesion is shown here:

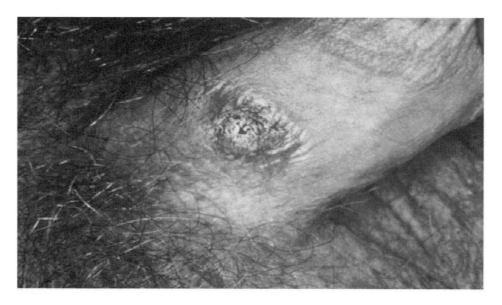

Which of the following is the <u>most</u> appropriate pharmacotherapy?

    A. Benzathine penicillin G 2.4 million units IM q week x 3
    B. Penicillin G 12 million units IV once daily for 10 days
    C. Procaine penicillin 4 million units IM x 1
    D. Benzathine penicillin G 2.4 million units IM
    E. Ceftriaxone 1 gram IM

224.

A 19-year-old college student presents with mild fever and cough. He has been coughing for several days and is not that ill. On physical examination, you note crackles in the left mid-lung fields.

Chest radiograph is as follows:

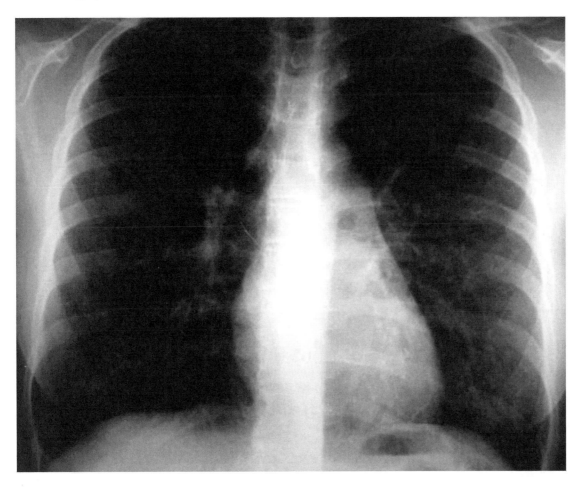

Which of the following is the <u>most</u> appropriate pharmacotherapy?

    A. Amoxicillin
    B. Amoxicillin-clavulanate
    C. Azithromycin
    D. Ceftriaxone
    E. Trimethoprim/sulfamethoxazole

225.

A 34-year-old man is brought to the emergency department in November with a painful rash on his hands and feet that began today. He has had fever and severe myalgias for one day. Three days ago, he had traveled to visit relatives in Texas. They had dogs that were known to have ticks, but he does not recall a tick bite. He is sexually active with the same partner for 14 years and denies any sexually transmitted diseases. He has never been tested for human immunodeficiency virus (HIV) infection.

Past Medical History: Asthma

Social History: Does not smoke. Drinks 3 beers on weekends.

Family History: Both parents alive and well. No siblings or children.

Review of symptoms: He denies headache, shortness of breath, or abdominal pain.

Physical Exam: BP 78/40 mmHg, PR 128, RR 24, Temp 101° F (38.3° C)
                HEENT: Bilateral large conjunctival hemorrhages
                Neck: Supple
                Nodes: None
                Heart: No murmurs or gallops
                Lungs: Clear to auscultation and percussion
                Abdomen: Bowel sounds normal, no organomegaly
                Extremities: Petechiae, purpura, and ecchymoses on the dorsal aspects of hands, wrists, feet, and ankles.

CBC: WBC 18,000, 54% polymorphonuclear, 18% bands, 8% monocytes, 20% lymphocytes. Hb 13.1 g/dL, platelets 53,000 mm^3
PT/INR: 17/2.26
PTT: 57s
D-dimer: 8.0
Creatinine: 2.8 mg/dL

A picture of the rash of the lower extremity is presented here:

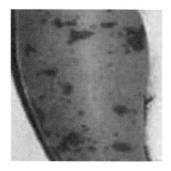

Which of the following is the <u>most</u> likely diagnosis?

   A. Secondary syphilis
   B. Toxic shock syndrome
   C. Rocky Mountain spotted fever
   D. Meningococcemia
   E. Gonococcemia

226.

A 21-year-old male with cystic fibrosis presents to your office with fever to 103° F (39.4° C), shortness of breath, and increased purulent sputum production. He has chills and appears to be quite ill. He has been hospitalized three times in the last 3 years for pneumonia exacerbation. In the past, MRSA and various strains of *Pseudomonas* were identified on bronchoscopy cultures. Physical exam reveals diffuse coarse breath sounds throughout. Chest radiograph reveals chronic scarring but is unchanged from his last radiograph. Sputum Gram stain reveals gram-positive cocci in clusters and large, gram-negative rods. Cultures are pending.

Which of the following is the **most** appropriate pharmacotherapy?

   A. None, because the organisms on Gram stain likely reflect colonization.
   B. Ampicillin and tobramycin.
   C. Vancomycin, tobramycin, and ceftazidime.
   D. Ciprofloxacin.
   E. Vancomycin, ceftriaxone, and tobramycin.

227.

A 28-year-old healthy man who lives in southern Missouri presents with 3 days of fever. He lives on a sheep, goat, and dairy farm. He has no lymphadenopathy, but has a slightly erythematous rash on his trunk. He likes to hunt with his brothers. He has removed numerous ticks from his body. His CBC shows a pancytopenia.

A bone marrow is performed and shows the following:

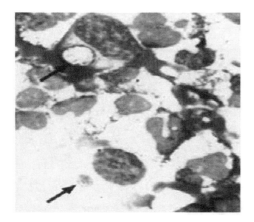

Which of the following is the **most** likely pathogen?

   A. *Ehrlichia*
   B. *Klebsiella*
   C. *Francisella*
   D. *Legionella*
   E. *Yersinia*

228.

The Office of Homeland Security notifies all physicians in your area that a possible bioterrorist event has occurred at a local high school football game. You are told to be on the lookout for people with pneumonia and a widened mediastinum on CXR. They tell you that these individuals will not be contagious via the respiratory route and will not require respiratory isolation.

Which of the following pathogens is <u>most</u> likely?

A. *Yersinia pestis*
B. *Bacillus anthracis*
C. Human herpesvirus 6
D. Smallpox virus

229.

A 20-year-old woman is evaluated in the emergency department for severe headache and altered consciousness. She undergoes a lumbar puncture, which reveals purulent CSF with a Gram stain showing intracellular gram-negative diplococci.

Of the following, who should receive meningococcal prophylaxis?

A. The third-year medical student who did the emergency department workup
B. The resident who did the lumbar puncture
C. The anesthesiologist who intubated the patient
D. All of the people listed

NEPHROLOGY

230.

A 77-year-old man arrives in the emergency department with complaints of nausea, vomiting, and general malaise. He has a long-standing history of hyperlipidemia, hypertension, and Type 2 diabetes mellitus. He has been a 1 pack/day smoker for the last 40 years. On physical exam, he is noted to be pale and stuporous. His blood pressure is 170/70, and his pulse is 88. He has loud carotid bruits, a faint systolic ejection murmur, clear lungs, and an obese abdomen that is soft and without peritoneal signs. Laboratory evaluation reveals a glucose of 142 mg/dL, potassium 5.4 mEq/L, creatinine 6.4 mg/dL, and BUN of 165 mg/dL. He has not had any urine output in the last 6 hours.

Which of the following is the best next step?

    A. Order ANCA and anti-GBM antibodies.
    B. Insert a temporary pacemaker in case hyperkalemia worsens.
    C. Obtain a CT of the abdomen and pelvis with contrast enhancement.
    D. Place a Foley catheter in the bladder.
    E. Place a temporary dual lumen dialysis catheter.

231.

A 77-year-old man has uremic symptomatology and is discovered to have 150 cc of urine in his bladder after catheterization. A digital rectal exam reveals a larger, firm prostate and heme-positive stool. An ultrasound demonstrates a single large, hyperechoic kidney with severe hydronephrosis. Further information from the patient is notable for a 20-lb weight loss over the last year and occasional night sweats. You are concerned the patient may have an obstructing intraabdominal mass, perhaps colon cancer, and you wish to perform a CT.

Which of the following is the best demonstrated strategy to reduce risk of contrast-associated nephrotoxicity?

    A. Begin high-dose furosemide and bicarbonate rich IV fluids.
    B. Administer normal saline IV until euvolemic.
    C. Begin high-dose furosemide, bicarbonate rich IV fluids, and n-acetylcysteine.
    D. Alternate furosemide, IV fluids, and mannitol.
    E. Give normal saline and furosemide to maintain equal ins and outs.

232.

Which of the following is a feature distinctive of Type 1 (distal) renal tubular acidosis?

    A. Hyperchloremic acidosis
    B. Associated with Fanconi syndrome
    C. Hyperkalemia
    D. Kidney stones
    E. Normal anion gap

233.

An 18-year-old boy is seen in your office during a "routine" pre-college physical. He has no chronic medical illness and does not use prescription or over-the-counter medications. His parents are worried because a maternal uncle had kidney failure at a young age and was on dialysis. On physical examination, he is in the 25th percentile for height and 25th percentile for weight; his blood pressure is 165/65 mmHg, and the remainder of his exam is normal with the exception of decreased high-frequency hearing bilaterally. The dipstick U/A reveals 2+ proteinuria and 10–15 RBCs/HPF. Repeat values 1 week and 1 month later continue to demonstrate dipstick positive proteinuria.

Which of the following will most likely establish a diagnosis?

A. Measurement of ANA and anti-double stranded DNA titers
B. Performance of an IVP and a renal ultrasound
C. Measurement of 24-hour urinary protein excretion
D. Measurement of supine and upright protein excretion
E. A kidney biopsy

234.

A 39-year-old woman with spina bifida is being evaluated for hematuria. She has a past history of urinary tract infections, but she has been healthy for the last year and is not on any new medications. She has no family history of kidney disease. On physical exam, her blood pressure is 102/60, and the rest of her exam is consistent with spina bifida, but otherwise unremarkable. On further evaluation, you note 10–15 RBCs/HPF but no casts or crystals. She has no proteinuria, and the serologic evaluation, including complements, ANCA and ANA, are all within normal limits. Urine calcium to creatinine ratio is 0.9. The ultrasound shows only one apparently normal appearing kidney without evidence for obstruction, and a urine culture returns with no growth.

Which of the following is the best management strategy at this time?

A. Start oxybutynin to prevent bladder spasms.
B. Push fluids, limit sodium intake, and maintain regular follow-up and vigilance for kidney stones.
C. Hospitalize and biopsy.
D. Empirically treat with antibiotics.
E. Perform an IVP or helical CT scan.

235.

A 42-year-old woman with a known history of severe steroid dependent asthma arrives in the emergency department with increasing respiratory distress over the last 8 hours. She has developed a low-grade fever and now is breathing at a rate of 30 breaths/min. Her pulse is 140 beats/min, and her blood pressure is 95/40 mmHg. She is becoming increasingly obtunded, unable to speak in full sentences, and has extensive use of her access muscles of respirations. A lung exam is notable for poor air exchange, decreased breath sounds in the left lung fields, and scattered expiratory and inspiratory wheezing. A stat arterial blood gas reveals: pH 7.1, pCO_2 50 mmHg, and HCO_3 15 mEq/L.

A basic metabolic panel is pending, but the available information is best described by which acid-base disorder?

A. Combined metabolic and respiratory acidosis
B. Metabolic acidosis alone
C. Metabolic acidosis with compensated respiratory alkalosis
D. Respiratory acidosis alone
E. Respiratory acidosis with compensated metabolic alkalosis

236.

A 56-year-old man now 2 years post-living related kidney transplant is admitted to the hospital with general malaise and a rising creatinine. His oral intake has been diminished over the last 2 weeks. He is somewhat evasive and unclear about his current medication use. On physical examination, the blood pressure is 105/65 mmHg; he is orthostatic; his abdomen is soft; and he has trace pretibial edema. On labs, his creatinine has risen from a baseline of 1.5 to 2.1 mg/dL over the last 6 months.

Which of the following is the appropriate immediate next step?

A. Perform a kidney biopsy.
B. Replete intravascular volume.
C. Transfuse packed red blood cells and give steroids.
D. Check and MRI of the renal artery.
E. Call the surgeon for possible exploration.

237.

A 34-year-old man returns to your office for a follow-up evaluation of persistent headaches, which began about one month ago. He reports a decrease in activity and some stumbling but a normal appetite. At the last visit you noted a blood pressure of 145/85. He has a prominent family history of hypertension, including two younger brothers. His past history has been otherwise unremarkable, and there are no new psychosocial issues or medications. His physical exam is completely normal again with the exception of a blood pressure of 160/95. You do some preliminary labs that are remarkable for a creatinine of 0.5 mg/dL and a potassium of 2.9 mEq/L.

Which of the following diagnoses is most consistent with this presentation?

A. Surreptitious laxative abuse
B. Liddle syndrome
C. Bartter syndrome
D. Gitelman syndrome
E. Nephrogenic DI

238.

When euvolemic patients are evaluated for persistent hyponatremia, which of the following is <u>not</u> considered in the differential diagnosis?

A. Syndrome of inappropriate antidiuresis
B. Chronic kidney disease
C. Hypercalcemia
D. Thyroid disease
E. Adrenal disease

239.

Spurious hyperkalemia may be due to:

A. Thrombocytosis
B. Leucopenia
C. Metabolic acidosis
D. Rhabdomyolysis
E. Hyperlipidemia

240.

A 29-year-old woman is admitted to the hospital for uncontrolled hypertension during the 29th week of her pregnancy. She is noted to have a blood pressure of 145/95, trace edema, and 3+ positive proteinuria on dipstick. Further laboratory analysis reveals a creatinine of 1.0 mg/dL, uric acid of 6.2 mg/dL, and a 24-hour urine protein collection of 1.5 gm.

Which of the following is the <u>most</u> appropriate next step in management?

A. Immediate delivery is indicated regardless of further laboratory testing.
B. Appropriate counseling should be offered for impending development of preeclampsia.
C. Magnesium in all forms should be avoided because of risk of toxicity.
D. Bed rest, antihypertensive therapy, and close monitoring of both the fetus and mother are appropriate at this stage.
E. ACE inhibitors are the drugs of choice in the setting of high-grade proteinuria.

241.

A 43-year-old woman is seen in your office for complaints of low back pain and dark urine. She is has had an unremarkable health history, and her only chronic problem has been diagnosed as fibromyalgia. She takes no medications and does <u>not</u> smoke. Her physical exam is unremarkable <u>except</u> for a BMI of 32. Her blood pressure is normal. Her back appears normal, and there is no tenderness or ability to elicit pain on examination. Of note is that a urine specimen appears "tea-colored" and is positive for blood and protein on dipstick. Microscopy reveals dysmorphic red blood cells and occasional red cell casts.

Which of the following is the <u>most</u> important next step in her care?

   A. Referral for kidney biopsy diagnosis
   B. Obtaining a 24-hour urine collection for protein
   C. Obtaining a spot urine protein to creatinine ratio
   D. Starting therapy with steroids
   E. Pushing hydration and repeating a U/A in a week or so

242.

A 68-year-old man has advanced chronic kidney disease due to obstructive uropathy and recurrent UTIs. He continues to have recurrent infections and was hospitalized last month with an *E. coli* pyelonephritis. He has refused surgery offered to correct his BPH. He now takes a daily dose of trimethoprim/sulfamethoxazole as UTI prophylaxis. On physical exam, you note mild hypertension but no other significant findings. His nephrologist, who saw him last week, has <u>not</u> referred him for transplantation but feels he will need dialysis in less than 6 months.

Which of the following reasons would explain a delay in transplantation in this man?

   A. He is too old.
   B. He has recurrent infections.
   C. He must not be on TMP/SMX within 12 months of a transplant.
   D. He is ineligible for transplant because of his hypertension.
   E. He must be on dialysis before getting a transplant.

243.

A 35-year-old woman begins to experience recurrent headaches at the start of a new job on Wall Street as a stock analyst. Her work performance has been excellent; her menses are regular and <u>not</u> associated with many of these headaches, and she takes no over-the-counter medications or prescription drugs. She does have a family history of hypertension and Type 2 diabetes mellitus. On physical, her BP is 188/110 (her records indicate she has had a normal BP on prior visits); she is tall and thin, and she has symmetric and strong pulses. Her cardiovascular exam is otherwise normal, and her lungs are clear; she has an otherwise unremarkable exam. An EKG reveals normal sinus rhythm at 66, and a BMP is notable for (standard units): Na 142, K 3.1, HCO_3 32, Cl 105, BUN 11, Creat 0.6, Gluc 95, Ca 9.8. A U/A is completely normal.

Which of the following diagnoses is <u>most</u> likely at this point?

   A. Coarctation of the aorta
   B. Primary hyperaldosteronism
   C. Cocaine use
   D. Stress of the new job and economic meltdown
   E. Fibromuscular dysplasia

244.

A 37-year-old obese man has been recently diagnosed with diabetes mellitus Type 2 and hypertension. He has a family history of ESRD and is very concerned he may end up on dialysis. You spend considerable time discussing weight loss, proper diet, and a healthy lifestyle.

In addition, to screen for microvascular disease and kidney disease in particular, which of the following is appropriate?

- A. You should screen for microalbuminuria now.
- B. You should wait 5 years before screening for microalbuminuria.
- C. The standard urine dipstick is sufficient for screening for diabetic kidney disease.
- D. Focus on weight loss and deal with the kidneys later.
- E. An eye exam will suffice to check for all microvascular disease.

245.

A 32-year-old new mother is brought to the emergency department by her family with palpitations and dizziness. She is noted to be hypervigilant and tachypneic with a respiratory rate of 28. She otherwise has a normal examination. Her labs are normal, <u>except</u> for an ABG. A blood gas is obtained and shows a pH =7.58, pCO_2 = 27, HCO_3 = 24. A-a gradient is calculated and is normal.

What is the <u>most</u> likely diagnosis?

- A. Acute fat emboli with pulmonary embolus
- B. Panic attack with respiratory alkalosis
- C. Occult laxative use
- D. Normal postpartum alkalosis
- E. Fear related to upcoming election cycle

246.

A 38-year-old man with known autosomal dominant polycystic kidney disease (PKD) has had a first episode of bleeding and a painful cyst. You have treated him as an inpatient with IV hydration and pain medications. He was adopted and unaware of his family history, but he thinks he had a kidney stone about 10 years ago. His blood pressure and pain are now well controlled, and he is ready for discharge. Because he is a new transfer to your care, you counsel him that he may suffer a number of renal and nonrenal complications from his PKD.

Which of the following complications should you inform him of with regard to his PKD?

A. Kidney manifestations may include recurrent flank pain, kidney stones, UTIs, and hematuria.
B. Mitral valve prolapse.
C. Intracranial aneurysms.
D. Diverticulosis and liver cysts.
E. All of the choices are complications of PKD.

247.

A surgical colleague asks for your opinion regarding prophylaxis for contrast-induced nephropathy in an elderly woman who has a creatinine of 2.5 mg/dL and is being considered for a contrast-enhanced CT of the chest and abdomen.

Which of the following pearls of advice do you offer your associate?

A. No special precautions are necessary for this level of kidney function.
B. A follow-up creatinine 12 hours after the procedure is sufficient to document no ill-effects.
C. Maintaining euvolemia with NS IVF is the single best strategy for prevention.
D. 2 weeks of n-acetylcysteine IV will nearly guarantee success.
E. An MRI with gadolinium is preferred.

248.

A 52-year-old male returns for follow-up from a recent emergency department visit where he was diagnosed to have a right-sided 4-mm kidney stone at the UPJ. He was advised to drink plenty of fluids, given pain medication, expect the stone to pass, and told to follow up with you in 2–3 days. He is irate that nothing more was done in the emergency department, including stone extraction.

What do you tell him during your visit today?

A. He should cut back on his milk and calcium intake because hypercalciuria is the most common metabolic abnormality associated with calcium-containing stones.
B. You will send him to the urologist today for stone extraction.
C. An increase in calcium intake paradoxically decreases risk of calcium containing stones.
D. He should avoid thiazide diuretics for the rest of his life.
E. Push fluids and eat more salt while he waits it out.

249.

You are asked to give advice to the ICU regarding therapy of a patient with pseudomonal sepsis.

Which of the following statements about aminoglycoside (AG) associated nephrotoxicity is true?

A. There is typically a time lag of 1–2 days after the start of therapy before clinical evidence of ATN begins to occur.
B. Nephrotoxicity is proportionate to the total dose of AG.
C. Coadministration of dopamine reduces the risk.
D. Other nephrotoxic agents increase the risk of ATN.
E. Both nephrotoxicity is proportionate to the total dose of aminoglycoside and other nephrotoxic agents increase the risk of ATN.

250.

During the routine evaluation of an established diabetic patient, urinalysis reveals a continued significant elevation of the urine microalbumin levels. The patient's blood pressure is well controlled at 122/78 mmHg, and the patient is otherwise asymptomatic. Her current medications include lisinopril 40 mg/day (max recommended dose).

Of the following, the <u>most</u> appropriate management decision would be:

A. Add verapamil.
B. Add an angiotensin receptor blocker.
C. Increase lisinopril to 80 mg/day.
D. Maintain current therapy and monitor BP.

251.

Rapid assessment of urine samples using dipstick indicators provides convenience and speed for many urinary concerns.

Urine dipsticks are <u>most</u> reliable for accurate results in which of the following situations?

A. Microalbumin assessment
B. Proteinuria with multiple myeloma
C. Proteinuria in minimal change disease
D. Urinary pH > 6.5
E. Urine specific gravity < 1.005

252.

A 34-year-old male presents with complaints of anxiety and "panic attacks" that occur 2–3 times per month. Physical exam is unremarkable, and the patient is referred for stress management. The patient returns one week later stating that symptoms are worsening, but, again, physical exam findings are normal. One week later the patient presents as a walk-in during one of his "attacks." On examination his pupils are constricted; his heart rate and blood pressure are elevated, and he is diaphoretic. He is <u>not</u> experiencing chest pains or shortness of breath. He indicates that this is typical of the episodes he has been experiencing.

Which of the following would be the <u>most</u> effective method of establishing the diagnosis in this situation?

    A. Abdominal CT scan
    B. Adrenal biopsy
    C. Ambulatory BP monitoring
    D. 24-hour urinary fractionated metanephrines

253.

A 32-year-old male presents with complaints of right-sided flank pain that started acutely during the night. Spiral CT shows a noncalcified obstructing lesion in the right distal ureter. He is admitted for analgesics and hydration. Early the next morning, the pain decreased, and he subsequently passed a piece of tissue.

Pathology on the specimen was consistent with renal papillary tissue and evaluation with IVP revealed a classic "ball in cup" pattern of the renal silhouette.

Of the following, which condition is <u>most</u> likely to have contributed to this pathology?

    A. Chronic analgesic abuse
    B. Excess vitamin C consumption
    C. Hepatitis C with cryoglobulinemia
    D. Right renal artery stenosis

254.

A 26-year-old female patient presents to your clinic with complaints of severe left-sided flank pain that started last evening and caused her to seek attention in the local urgent care clinic. She was diagnosed with a kidney stone and was sent home on analgesics and oral hydration. The pain is significantly improved today. The patient asks what caused the stone and what specific steps she can institute to prevent recurrences.

In order to best answer her concerns, an accurate diagnosis of the stone type is desired. The best way to identify her type of kidney stone is:

    A. Serum tests for calcium, uric acid, electrolytes, and phosphate
    B. 24-hour urine collection for calcium, oxalate, uric acid, phosphate, and magnesium
    C. Family history of kidney stones or metabolic diseases
    D. Microscopic crystal evaluation of the renal stone

255.

You are asked to evaluate a new patient in the area presenting with hematuria. As part of the evaluation, laboratory studies are requested, including urinalysis, cultures, and complement levels.

Which of the following glomerulonephropathies is <u>most</u> likely to demonstrate normal complement studies?

    A. IgA nephropathy
    B. Lupus glomerulonephritis
    C. Membranoproliferative glomerulonephritis
    D. Post-streptococcal glomerulonephritis

256.

A 44-year-old male with recent bariatric intervention returns for follow-up after having passed a kidney stone 4 weeks previously. The stone was identified as a calcium oxalate stone. He is requesting information to help reduce his risk for recurrence.

Which of the following would be <u>most</u> likely to reduce the risk for recurrent oxalate stones in this patient?

    A. High-dose vitamin C supplements
    B. A low-calcium diet
    C. Citrate supplements
    D. Low dose furosemide daily

257.

A 36-year-old female presents with complaints of increased frequency, urgency, and intermittent dysuria. She states that she has seen multiple physicians in the past and previous evaluation has noted occasional microscopic hematuria. Urine cultures in the past have been consistently normal. She denies any history of STD or vaginal discharge. Her menstrual periods are regular and do <u>not</u> seem to affect the symptoms.

The physical examination today is within normal limits including blood pressure and pelvic exam. Complete blood cell counts demonstrate no evidence of anemia.

The patient insists that some action be taken to address her symptoms.

Which of the following would be <u>most</u> appropriate at this time to help determine the problem?

    A. Perform random serial urine cultures.
    B. Prescribe an anxiolytic agent.
    C. Prescribe topical estrogen.
    D. Prophylactic dosages of antibiotics.
    E. If performed in the past, get results of prior urinalysis, urine culture, and postvoid residual.

258.

A 34-year-old female with end-stage renal disease and chronic abdominal peritoneal dialysis (CAPD) presents to the emergency department with complaints of diffuse abdominal pain over the preceding 12 hours. She has noted significant clouding to the dialysate over the course of the day.

On examination, she has diffuse tenderness to abdominal palpation and has rebound pain across the entire abdomen.

Which of the following is true regarding CAPD-related peritonitis?

A. CAPD peritonitis is typically a multi-organism infection.
B. Enteric organisms predominate as the etiological agents.
C. Centrifuged dialysate grown in blood culture medium improves the yield.
D. IV antibiotics are the primary treatment modality.
E. Peritonitis is a contraindication to introducing fluids into the abdominal cavity.

259.

A 34-year-old man is brought to the emergency department by EMS after being found obtunded in a drainage ditch. He lives with his wife and is unemployed. His wife reports that he drinks 6–8 beers per night and smokes cigarettes but does not use any drugs.

PE: 100/70, HR 125, RR 22
He is obtunded with a normal funduscopic exam, clear lungs, and normal heart sounds. His abdomen is soft. He moves all his extremities.
Na 138, K 4.6, Cl 107, HCO_3 12
Glucose 88, Creat 1.1, BUN 8
U/A 1.015, pH 5.5
UDS negative; no measurable ethanol
SOsm 355

Which of the following is the most likely diagnosis?

A. Acute aspirin overdose
B. Isopropyl alcohol ingestion
C. Methanol ingestion
D. Non-ketotic hyperosmolar coma
E. Diabetic ketoacidosis

260.

An 80-year-old man with long-standing diabetes and HTN is admitted with severe low back pain and increasing confusion. He has a 3-month history of 20-lb weight loss and no prior history of kidney disease. On examination, he is frail and generally decompensated with normal vital signs and point tenderness over L3.
Na 139, K 5.9, Cl 115, HCO_3 18
BUN 68, Creat 3.6, Ca 11.1, Glu 145
U/A 1.020, pH 6.0, 2 RBCs/HPF, trace protein
24-hour urine: clearance 18 cc/m; protein 5.5 gm

Which of the following is the <u>most</u> appropriate next step in patient care?

A. Hepatitis serologies
B. PSA
C. Colonoscopy
D. Urine and serum electrophoresis
E. Urine for Hansel's stain for eosinophils and cytology

261.

A 77-year-old man arrives in the emergency department with complaints of nausea, vomiting, and general malaise. He has <u>not</u> had any urine output in the last 6 hours.

PMH: Hyperlipidemia, hypertension, and Type 2 diabetes mellitus, tobacco abuse x 40 years

Exam: Pale and stuporous
BP 170/70, HR 88
Loud carotid bruits
A faint systolic ejection murmur
Clear lungs
Obese abdomen that is soft and without peritoneal signs
Labs:
Glu 142 mg/dL
K 5.4 mEq/L
Creatinine 6.4 mg/dL
BUN 165 mg/dL

Which of the following is the next best step in management?

A. Order ANCA and anti-GBM antibodies.
B. Insert a temporary pacemaker in case hyperkalemia worsens.
C. Obtain a CT of the abdomen and pelvis with contrast enhancement.
D. Place a Foley catheter in the bladder.
E. Place a temporary dual lumen dialysis catheter.

262.

A 64-year-old woman with a past history of hypertension, hyperlipidemia, and osteoarthritis presents complaining of lower extremity edema. Recent history includes an ophthalmologic referral by her optometrist for laser surgery of an inexplicable proliferative retinopathy.

Meds: Ibuprofen 400 mg bid prn arthritic pain, metoprolol, simvastatin

Exam: BP 122/74, HR 82
Fundi <u>not</u> visible, abdomen is morbidly obese. 3+ pitting edema of the lower extremities to mid-calf.

Labs:
Fasting BMP: Creat 1.1 mg/dL, glu 135 mg/dL
U/A: 3+ glucose and 4+ protein

Of the following laboratory findings, which supports the <u>most</u> likely diagnosis?

    A. A positive c-ANCA
    B. A 24-hour urine total protein of 8.5 gm
    C. M spike on a serum protein electrophoresis
    D. A creatinine clearance of 140 mL/min
    E. A positive HBsAg

263.

A severely mentally retarded 46-year-old male is brought to the emergency department by neighbors after he was found down in his garage. He is obtunded, and his clothing is soiled with stool and urine. He is afebrile. Orthostatic vital signs show a change in blood pressure and pulse between lying and sitting. Kussmaul respirations are noted. Neurologic exam is non-focal.

Na 133, K 2.5, Cl 118, HCO_3 5
BUN 52, Creat 3.4
U/A: pH 5.0
Urine Na 6
ABG: pH 7.25, pCO_2 20, HCO_3 5

What is the acid-base abnormality?

    A. HAGMA
    B. NAGMA
    C. HAGMA + respiratory acidosis
    D. HAGMA + respiratory alkalosis
    E. Metabolic alkalosis

264.

A 29-year-old presents with severe abdominal pain and renal cysts by U/S.

Which of the following associated conditions is <u>most</u> likely to be observed with this patient's underlying diagnosis?

    A. Pancreatic cancer
    B. Neurofibromas
    C. Phenylketonuria
    D. Cerebral aneurysms
    E. Testicular torsion

ENDOCRINOLOGY

265.

A 24-year-old female with Graves disease was treated with radioactive iodine 9 months ago. Her weight has returned to normal; she no longer has palpitations or heat intolerance, and her menstrual periods are regular. Thyroid function studies last week revealed a free T_4 of 1.4 (0.9–1.5) and a TSH of < 0.05 (0.2–4.2).

Which of the following should you recommend now?

A. Methimazole
B. Another dose of radioactive iodine
C. Measure TSH receptor antibody
D. No intervention

266.

A 70-year-old man with steroid-dependent asthma is admitted with fever, congestive heart failure, atrial fibrillation, and episodes of confusion. On exam, his thyroid is smooth and three times enlarged. His free T_4 is 6.3 (0.9–1.5), and his TSH is suppressed. In the ICU, he has received intravenous beta-blocker therapy and 100 mg of hydrocortisone.

What is the most important next step in treating the hyperthyroidism?

A. Administer radioactive iodine.
B. Administer methimazole.
C. Administer cold iodine.
D. Arrange for a technetium scan.

267.

A 50-year-old male has a 1-month history of tremor, palpitations, heat intolerance, and hyperdefecation. He has no history of thyroid disease, but his sister takes thyroid hormone. His pulse is 100; his thyroid is tender to palpation and mildly enlarged and non-nodular. He has no proptosis. A free T_4 is 2.1 (0.9–1.5) and TSH is 0.01 (0.2–4.2). A serum thyroglobulin level is elevated.

What is the most likely explanation for the elevated free T_4?

A. Graves disease
B. Surreptitious use of thyroid hormone
C. Subacute thyroiditis
D. Toxic multinodular goiter

268.

A 68-year-old woman has lost 15 pounds and has fatigue. There is a 2-cm nodule in the thyroid; pulse is 90; the skin is dry; and there is a mild tremor of the outstretched hands. A free T_4 is 1.9 (0.9–1.5) and TSH is < 0.05 (0.2–4.2).

What is the next <u>most</u> appropriate step in evaluating the nodule?

    A. Technetium scan
    B. Ultrasound guided fine needle aspiration
    C. Measure TSH receptor antibodies
    D. Measure T_3

269.

A 30-year-old male has gained 30 pounds, developed muscle weakness, hypertension, and bruising. After an overnight dexamethasone suppression test, his 8 a.m. cortisol was 15. Last week an 8 a.m. ACTH was 1 (10–60). Urine free cortisol levels measured before and after 2 and 8 mg of dexamethasone were:

    baseline   1,400 µg
    2 mg   1,300 µg
    8 mg   1,200 µg

What is the <u>most</u> likely etiology of the glucocorticoid excess in this patient?

    A. Pituitary adenoma
    B. Adrenal adenoma
    C. Ectopic ACTH syndrome
    D. Hypothyroidism

270.

A 17-year-old boy presents with a 1-year history of breast enlargement and no other complaints. His height is 71 inches; he weighs 170 pounds; his testes measure ~ 1 cm; the thyroid is <u>not</u> palpable, and there is bilateral palpable breast tissue. Testosterone is 190 (280–800); ß-HCG is negative; FSH is 30 (2–12); LH 25 (4–15); and estradiol is 10 (20–80).

What is the <u>most</u> likely cause of his breast enlargement?

    A. Klinefelter syndrome
    B. Prolactinoma
    C. Testicular tumor
    D. Nonfunctioning pituitary tumor

271.

A 20-year-old female is referred for treatment of facial hair, which has been present since age 12. Her menstrual periods are regular; her BMI is 20. She has dark hair on the upper lip, cheeks, and areolae, and her pelvic exam is normal. Her A1c is 5.1%, and her testosterone level is 20 (6–82).

What should you recommend now?

    A. Measure 17-hydroxyprogesterone.
    B. Transvaginal ultrasound.
    C. Begin metformin.
    D. Begin spironolactone.

272.

A 24-year-old female has had no menstrual periods for 15 months and has dark hair on her face, chest, lip, breasts, and lower abdomen. Her pelvic exam shows an enlarged clitoris. Testosterone is 220 (6–82); DHEA-S 200 (200–335); and her A1c is 7.8%.

Which of the following is the <u>most</u> likely cause of the hirsutism?

    A. Polycystic ovarian syndrome
    B. Ovarian tumor
    C. Idiopathic hirsutism
    D. Congenital adrenal hyperplasia
    E. Adrenal tumor

273.

A 40-year-old female has lost 10 pounds over the last 2 months, complains of excessive thirst, and has repeated vaginal yeast infections. Her BMI is 23, and her exam is normal <u>except</u> for dry buccal mucosa and vaginal discharge. Her fasting blood sugar this morning is 380.

Which of the following would you recommend as initial therapy for the diabetes?

    A. Metformin
    B. Glipizide
    C. Insulin
    D. Pioglitazone

274.

A 27-year-old woman with Type 1 diabetes is taking 15 units of NPH and 10 units of regular insulin before breakfast and around 6 p.m. She cannot afford a more expensive insulin preparation. Her exam is normal, and the table below is a record of her blood sugars recorded at home. At least once per week, she awakens around 3 a.m. with hypoglycemia.

	3 A.M.	FASTING	LUNCH	SUPPER	BEDTIME
Day 1	90	240	140	110	120
Day 2	100	220	130	120	140

Which of the following adjustments will improve her blood sugar control?

A. Increase the a.m. regular insulin to 15 units.
B. Increase the p.m. NPH to 20 units.
C. Move the p.m. NPH to bedtime.
D. Move her p.m. regular to bedtime.

275.

A 75-year-old man presents with visual loss. He has cold intolerance, fatigue, weight gain, and headaches. His exam shows B/P 110/60, pale skin, ↓ beard growth, and breast enlargement. Lab shows prolactin 24, cortisol 2 (↓), testosterone 50 (↓), and free T_4 0.4 (↓).

Replacement therapy is initiated, and he is scheduled for formal visual fields.

What is the next step?

A. Neurosurgery consult.
B. Radiation therapy consult.
C. Cabergoline.
D. Measure GH and IGF-1.

276.

After an extremely difficult delivery of her second child, a 26-year-old female developed persistent amenorrhea and is now taking estrogen and progesterone. In the last 6 months, she has noted constipation, fatigue, dry skin, and her weight has increased by 10 pounds. Thyroid function studies revealed free T_4 0.6 (0.8–1.9) and TSH 0.6 (0.2–4.2).

What is the most appropriate next step?

A. Start levothyroxine.
B. Measure T_3.
C. Technetium scan.
D. Serum cortisol.

277.

A 30-year-old woman complains of increased thirst and nocturia. She has a normal exam, and her electrolytes, calcium, and glucose are normal. Following an overnight fast, her urine specific gravity was 1.020, and her urine osmolality was 700.

What should you do now?

A. H_2O deprivation test.
B. Begin amiloride.
C. Begin DDAVP®.
D. Reassurance.

278.

A 75-year-old female has been taking 1 grain (60 mg) of Thyroid-S Armour® thyroid extract daily for 15 years and feels great. She won't take any other type of thyroid medication. Today her free T_4 is 0.5 (0.9–1.7), TSH 1.2 (0.2–4.2), and T_3 2.3 (0.8–2). Her exam (including the thyroid exam) is normal.

Which of the following should you recommend?

A. Increase dose to 1½ grains.
B. Make no changes.
C. Measure free T_3.
D. Measure antithyroid antibodies.

279.

A 25-year-old female nursing assistant has a 2-month history of palpitations. She is trying to lose weight. On exam, her thyroid is <u>not</u> palpable, and she has a fine tremor.
FT_4 2.1 (↑), TSH 0.01 (↓), thyroglobulin (↓)

What is the <u>most</u> likely diagnosis?

A. Graves
B. Surreptitious use of thyroid hormone
C. Subacute thyroiditis
D. Hot nodule

280.

An 80-year-old man has been hospitalized for 1 month after treatment of a perforated ulcer. He has no history of thyroid disease. Over the last week, he has noted cold intolerance, dry skin, and periorbital puffiness. His surgeons obtained a FT_4↓, TSH↓, and T3↓.

You are asked to treat the hypothyroidism.

What do you recommend?

A. 0.025 mg levothyroxine.
B. 10 µg liothyronine.
C. Repeat FT_4, TSH and T_3 in one week.
D. No intervention.

281.

A 36-year-old woman has gained 20 pounds, has high blood pressure, and many bruises. Her BMI is 30. Her only medication is a BCP. A serum cortisol drawn at 8 a.m. after 1 mg of dex at 11 p.m. was 10 ($\uparrow$).

What should you do next?

A. No further therapy.
B. Do a 24-hr urine cortisol.
C. Measure ACTH.
D. Do an 8 mg dexamethasone suppression test.

282.

A 50-year-old woman has gained 50 pounds and bruises easily. She has a buffalo hump, proximal muscle weakness, and pale striae on her abdomen. A 24-hr urine cortisol is 25 (< 50).

Which of the following is correct?

A. She likely has pituitary Cushing's.
B. She likely has an adrenal adenoma.
C. The next step is to measure ACTH.
D. Cushing's has been excluded.

283.

A 32-year-old was recently diagnosed with Addison disease. For 1 month she has taken 5 mg of prednisone daily and feels better. Her only other medication is levothyroxine. Labs today showed sodium 130, potassium 4.9, and CO_2 20.

What should you do now?

A. Check cortisol and ACTH.
B. Change prednisone to hydrocortisone.
C. Do adrenal CT scan.
D. Increase dose of prednisone.

284.

A 60-year-old has fatigue, weight loss, abdominal pain, and loss of axillary hair. His cortisol is 1.2 and stimulated to 5 after Cortrosyn®. You start 5 mg of prednisone. However, his symptoms do <u>not</u> improve, and he has cold intolerance and constipation. His TSH is 0.9 (nl).

What should you do?

    A. Increase prednisone to 10 mg daily.
    B. Add fludrocortisone.
    C. Measure testosterone.
    D. Measure free T_4.

285.

A 29-year-old female presents for evaluation of fatigue. She reports decreased energy throughout the day that has progressively worsened over the past 2 months. She notes occasional palpitations and 7-kg weight loss. She denies any recent illness or infection. On physical exam, her HR is 95, and her BP is 145/87. Thyroid exam reveals a smooth, enlarged thyroid gland that is nontender to palpation.

Thyroid function testing reveals
TSH – < 0.01 uU/mL (0.5–5.0 uU/mL)
Free T_4 – 2.6 ng/dL (0.9–2.4 ng/dL)

Radioactive iodine uptake scan reveals decreased uptake throughout the thyroid gland.

Which of the following is the <u>most</u> likely diagnosis?

    A. Chronic lymphocytic thyroiditis
    B. Subacute thyroiditis
    C. Toxic multinodular goiter
    D. Graves disease
    E. Exogenous hyperthyroidism

286.

A 26-year-old female presents for evaluation of neck pain and fatigue. She described the pain as located in the front of her neck and does <u>not</u> radiate, but has been constant over the last week. She reports she recently had an upper respiratory infection with cough, nasal congestion, sore throat, and fever last month. Review of systems elicits that the patient has felt fatigue over the last 2–3 weeks as well. On physical exam, her HR is 95, and her BP is 145/87. HEENT exam reveals a clear oropharynx and nares. Thyroid exam reveals a smooth, enlarged thyroid gland that is exquisitely tender to palpation. The remainder of the physical exam is unremarkable.

Thyroid function testing reveals
TSH – < 0.01 uU/mL (0.5–5.0 uU/mL)
Free T_4 – 2.6 ng/dL (0.9–2.4 ng/dL)

Radioactive iodine uptake scan reveals decreased uptake throughout the thyroid gland.

Which of the following is the <u>most</u> likely diagnosis?

    A. Chronic lymphocytic thyroiditis
    B. Subacute thyroiditis
    C. Toxic multinodular goiter
    D. Graves disease
    E. Medullary thyroid carcinoma

287.

A 26-year-old female presents for evaluation of neck pain and fatigue. She describes the pain as located in the front of her neck and does <u>not</u> radiate, but has been constant over the last week. She reports she recently had an upper respiratory infection with cough, nasal congestion, sore throat, and fever last month. Review of systems elicits that the patient has felt fatigue over the last 2–3 weeks as well. On physical exam, her HR is 95, and her BP is 145/87. HEENT exam reveals a clear oropharynx and nares. Thyroid exam reveals a smooth, enlarged thyroid gland that is exquisitely tender to palpation. The remainder of the physical exam is unremarkable.

Thyroid function testing reveals
TSH – < 0.01 uU/mL (0.5–5.0 uU/mL)
Free T_4 – 2.6 ng/dL (0.9–2.4 ng/dL)

Radioactive iodine uptake scan reveals decreased uptake throughout the thyroid gland.

Which of the following statements regarding the prognosis of the disease is <u>most</u> accurate?

    A. The patient will likely require radioiodine ablation.
    B. Additional imaging would help to direct management.
    C. The patient will likely require thyroid hormone replacement in the future.
    D. The patient is at risk for relapse of symptoms.
    E. No additional therapy is needed.

288.

Following testing for lipid levels, the results for a 28-year-old male are consistent with the diagnosis of type I hyperlipoproteinemia.

Which of the following is the <u>most</u> likely consequence of this condition?

    A. Glomerulonephritis
    B. Pancreatitis
    C. Cholecystitis
    D. Coronary vascular disease

289.

A 72-year-old female presents to the emergency department with increasing lethargy following two days of increasing nausea and vomiting. She was diagnosed with a urinary tract infection three days ago and started on a course of oral ciprofloxacin. Her past history is remarkable for a diagnosis of temporal arteritis six months previously for which she has recently completed an extended weaning for oral dexamethasone.

On examination, her blood pressure is 112/65 mmHg: temperature is 97.5° F (36.4° C); heart rate 92/min, and respiratory rate 14 breaths/min. She rouses with stimulation and follows simple commands. There is no meningismus and no costovertebral angle tenderness.

Urinalysis shows 3–5 RBC and trace protein but is otherwise unremarkable. CBC shows white blood cell count of $9.8 \times 10^3/mm^3$ with a normal differential.

Of the following, the __most__ important intervention at this time would be:

A. Broad-spectrum IV antibiotics
B. IV bolus of normal saline
C. CT scan of the head
D. Drug screen
E. IV hydrocortisone

290.

A 27-year-old male presents with renal colic and is found to have nephrolithiasis. The stone is noted to be composed of calcium phosphate. His only medications are a thiazide diuretic and megadose vitamin supplements. After the acute episodes have resolved, an evaluation is instituted and discovers an elevated serum ionized calcium of 3.6 mmol/L (1.1–1.4 mmol/L). A parathyroid hormone (PTH) level of 120 pg/mL (10–65 pg/mL) was obtained.

Which of the following is the __most__ consistent with this clinical presentation?

A. Hyperthyroidism
B. MEN Type I
C. Thiazide diuretic
D. Vitamin D intoxication

291.

During the routine evaluation of a 37-year-old female, you note a palpable lesion in the right lobe of the thyroid. The patient has been asymptomatic and was unaware of the lesion. It is firm and mobile, with distinct borders. No other lesions or abnormalities are detected.

Which of the following would be the __most__ appropriate next step in the evaluation of this nodule?

A. TSH
B. Fine needle aspiration
C. Thyroid ultrasound
D. Thyroid scan

292.

During routine laboratory screening for an asymptomatic healthy adult, the following lipid values were obtained:

Cholesterol

Total	222	mg/dL	< 200	Desirable
			200–239	Borderline high
			≥ 240	High
LDL	137	mg/dL	< 100	Optimal
			100–129	Near or above normal
			130–159	Borderline High
			160–189	High
			≥ 190	Very High
HDL	75	mg/dL	< 40	Low
			≥ 60	High
Triglycerides	1,820	mg/dL	< 150	

Based on these laboratory findings, which of the following abnormalities would be the <u>most</u> likely complication?

A. Pancreatitis
B. Hypernatremia
C. Xanthelasmata
D. Nephrotic syndrome
E. Hepatic cirrhosis

293.

A 62-year-old woman comes to clinic with diarrhea for 3 weeks. The patient began having nonbloody diarrhea three weeks ago. She has 4–5 soft bowel movements per day. She has no abdominal pain, nausea, or vomiting. Over the same time, she has developed fatigue and has become anxious about work and her family.
On review of systems, she complains of palpitations.

She has a past medical history of hypertension and hyperlipidemia and coronary artery disease.
Medications include aspirin, simvastatin, hydrochlorothiazide, and lisinopril.

On physical exam her heart rate is 110; blood pressure is 148/89, and she is anxious appearing. Her heart exam shows tachycardia, and no murmurs, rubs, or gallops. Her lung and abdominal exam is unremarkable. She has a resting tremor, and her reflexes are brisk.

Blood testing shows an undetectably low TSH and elevated T_4 and T_3.

What is the next step in the management of this patient?

A. Begin propranolol.
B. Order a radioactive iodine uptake scan.
C. Refer to endocrinology.
D. Order a thyroid-stimulating antibody panel.

294.

A 62-year-old man presents with muscle aches and fatigue. Over the last 1 month he has been having more pain with movement, especially in his thighs and upper arms. He has difficulty getting out of a chair without using his arms. He has never had similar symptoms in the past, and he denies oral ulcers, hair loss, skin rash, swollen, or painful joints.

His past medical history is significant for coronary artery disease with 2 myocardial infarctions and multiple stents placed. He has a history of hypertension, diabetes, and hyperlipidemia. His medications include atorvastatin, metoprolol, lisinopril, clopidogrel, metformin, aspirin, and gemfibrozil.

On physical exam, his blood pressure is 120/78; pulse is 65. His exam is significant for muscle tenderness of his thighs and upper arms. He has no rash, joint swelling, or joint pain.
Laboratory testing reveals a creatine kinase (CK) of 750 IU/L (normal is 60–400 IU/L). You diagnose statin-induced myositis, and stop his atorvastatin and gemfibrozil. His CK normalizes; however, his LDL rises to 190.

What is the next step in management of his hyperlipidemia?

A. Restart atorvastatin, follow CK, and titrate dose.
B. Start a bile-acid sequestrant.
C. Begin ezetimibe.
D. Begin pravastatin, follow CK, and titrate dose.

295.

You are called to evaluate a 55-year-old insulin-dependent diabetic woman with acute mental status changes during her hospitalization for lower extremity cellulitis. The nurse reports that during her last vital sign check, the patient was unable to verbalize answers to questions and appeared to be very agitated. On exam she is afebrile, BP 140/87, HR 95, RR 22, and 98% O_2 saturation. General exam shows the patient to be diaphoretic and somewhat pale. Heart exam reveals RRR without murmur or gallop. Lungs clear. Left lower extremity is tender to palpation without fluctuance with an area of erythema that has not spread beyond the marked area drawn at the time of admission.

What is the next best step in the management of this patient?

A. ECG
B. Capillary blood glucose
C. Emergent surgical consultation
D. 25 gm IV 50% dextrose
E. 1 mg SC glucagon

296.

A 55-year-old man with past history of hypertension and diabetes is admitted for abdominal pain. His home medications are lisinopril, amlodipine, metformin, and glipizide. Overnight the patient becomes diaphoretic, and his wife reports to the nurse that he has been very irritable since missing his dinner meal tray to undergo diagnostic imaging to evaluate his pain. He is on IV fluids of 1/2 normal saline. On exam, the patient's vital signs are: temperature 37° C, BP 140/87, HR 95, RR 22, and 98% O_2 saturation. He is difficult to arouse and does <u>not</u> verbally respond to questions. A bedside capillary blood glucose measurement is measured to be 45 mg/dL.

What is the next best step in the management of this patient?

    A. 25 gm IV 50% dextrose
    B. 1 mg SC glucagon
    C. 15 gm of oral carbohydrate replacement
    D. Discontinue metformin
    E. Discontinue glipizide

297.

A 47-year-old febrile, diabetic man presents to the emergency department after being found down by his wife. Initial evaluation reveals a left lower lobe pneumonia.

Admission labs: Na 128, K 3.2, Cl 98, HCO_3 7, Glu 700

He is given 2 L of 0.9% NaCl, a bolus of insulin, and started on a continuous insulin infusion.

Repeat labs: Na 136, K 3.0, Cl 105, HCO_3 19, Glu 375

Which of the following is the <u>most</u> appropriate next step with regard to insulin and IVFs?

    A. Change to 5% dextrose with 0.45% NaCl and continue the insulin infusion at the current rate.
    B. Give 10 U regular insulin, stop the IVF and the insulin infusion, and allow the patient to eat.
    C. Give 10 U regular insulin, stop the IVF, continue the insulin infusion for 2 hours at the current rate, then stop.
    D. Continue the current IVF and double the insulin infusion rate.
    E. Continue the current management.

298.

A 32-year-old woman presented to the emergency department with pain in the RUQ, fever, and jaundice. She was diagnosed with ascending cholangitis and admitted to the ICU. After stabilizing, her heart rate was recorded as 55–65 bpm for the past 2 days. Thyroid studies were ordered with the following results:

TSH: 0.20 (0.5–5.0), Free T_4: 1.7 (5–12)

You are consulted for recommendations on the need for further evaluation and institution of thyroid replacement hormone.

Which of the following is the <u>most</u> appropriate next step in patient care?

    A. Diagnose secondary hypothyroidism and order an MRI of the pituitary.
    B. Start levothyroxine 100 micrograms daily.
    C. Start levothyroxine 50 micrograms daily.
    D. Reassure the consulting physician.
    E. Order a thyroid uptake scan.

299.

A 49-year-old man presents to your clinic with a 4-month history of cold intolerance, easy fatigue, depression, some weight gain, and constipation.

FT_4: 0.5 (0.8–1.8)

TSH: 0.5 (0.5–4.0)

Which of the following is the <u>most</u> likely diagnosis?

    A. Hashimoto disease
    B. Primary hypothyroidism
    C. Secondary hypothyroidism
    D. Euthyroid sick syndrome
    E. No thyroid disease

300.

A 47-year-old man comes to your clinic for a pre-employment physical. He denies any PMH. His BMI is 31. PE is unremarkable. Labs reveal a fasting plasma glucose of 128 mg/dL.

Which of the following is the <u>most</u> appropriate next step in patient care?

    A. Diagnose him with prediabetes.
    B. Diagnose him with diabetes.
    C. Diagnose him with chemical diabetes.
    D. Recheck a fasting blood glucose on a different day.

301.

A 58-year-old woman comes in for follow-up. She was diagnosed with DM 6 months ago by the cardiologist, who is following her for Stage 3 CHF (stable). She follows an AHA diet, takes her medications, and follows her walking program.

Meds: metformin 500 mg qhs

Blood glucose levels:
Fasting 100–140
Postprandial 200–240
Bedtime 100–120

HbA1c: 8.5%
Creatinine: 1.5 mg/dL

Spot urine albumin: creatinine 20
BMI: 30.5 kg/m^2

Which of the following is the <u>most</u> appropriate next step in patient care?

    A. Stop metformin and start either repaglinide or nateglinide.
    B. Increase metformin to 1,000 mg bid in steps as tolerated.
    C. Add pioglitazone to metformin.
    D. Add acarbose or miglitol to metformin.
    E. Stop metformin and start pioglitazone.

302.

Your patient is clinically hyperthyroid and has a slight nontender goiter.

Free T$_4$ 2.2 (0.9–1.8)
TSH 0.25 (0.5–5.0)
Nuclear scan: homogeneous pattern
Uptake 4% (↓)

Which of the following is the <u>most</u> likely diagnosis?

    A. Graves disease
    B. Subacute thyroiditis
    C. Silent thyroiditis
    D. Exogenous T$_4$
    E. Toxic multinodular goiter

303.

Your patient is a 45-year-old male whose father died of an MI at age 57. He does <u>not</u> smoke and is <u>not</u> on any medication.

BP 120/72
HDL 42 mg/dL

What is his target LDL?

    A. < 190
    B. < 160
    C. < 130
    D. < 100
    E. < 70

304.

A 46-year-old female with a history of diabetes presents obtunded. She has no other medical problems and lives with her 17-year-old daughter. She takes NPH insulin bid. Her daughter states that recently, the patient has been having severe nightmares but otherwise has been in her usual state of health. She underwent menopause from age 38–42.

PE: T 96° F, BP 110/60, HR 66, RR 14
Alopecia on the head, pubic region, and eyebrows
Arousable to deep sternal rub, reactive pupils
Delayed reflexes

Na 122
K 3.4
Cl 82
HCO_3 23
Glu 110
BUN 40
Creat 1.0
Hgb 10.6
MCV 86
TSH 0.45 (0.5–5.0)
Free T_4 0.75 (0.9–2.4)
FSH 15 (> 35 postmenopausal)
LH 22 (> 30 postmenopausal)

Which of the following is the <u>most</u> likely diagnosis?

    A. Primary adrenal insufficiency
    B. Insulin overdose
    C. Primary hypothyroidism
    D. Pituitary insufficiency
    E. Carbon monoxide poisoning

305.

A 48-year-old woman comes to your clinic with fatigue and galactorrhea. Thin white fluid can be expressed from each breast. She has no breast masses or tenderness. Her skin is dry. Recent mammogram was normal.

Prolactin level: 40 (1.4–14.2)
MRI: 8-mm pituitary mass

Which of the following is the next best step in management?

    A. Refer her to a neurosurgeon for resection of a prolactinoma.
    B. Start bromocriptine.
    C. Recheck prolactin level in 6–12 months.
    D. Check TSH.
    E. Look for an unknown nonpituitary cancer.

306.

You are asked to see a 48-year-old Caucasian male who was admitted to the ICU for hypotension after an MVA, when he suffered a broken thumb. The orthopedic surgeon reported a simple fracture and placed a cast on his hand, but the patient lost consciousness a few minutes later and was noted to have a BP of 75/palp. BP is 100/64 while on IV saline.

HR in the ER was 130 but is now 80. Temp is 98.7° F.
You note that he is thin and tan with sparse axillary hair. His skin is warm and moist. He denies fatigue or cold intolerance.

Na 134
K 5.6
Cl 102
HCO$_3$ 22
BUN 42
Creat 0.7
Glu 61
Head CT normal

Which of the following is the <u>most</u> appropriate next step in patient care?

    A. Hydrocortisone.
    B. Hydrocortisone + fludrocortisone and order an ACTH stimulation test.
    C. Dexamethasone + fludrocortisone and order an ACTH stimulation test.
    D. Thyroxine daily.
    E. Hydrocortisone and thyroxine daily. Order an ACTH stimulation test and TSH.

HEMATOLOGY

307.

An 82-year-old woman presents to her local emergency department with complaints of a mass under her tongue. Evaluation reveals it to be a large hematoma, and she is sent home with instructions to use local measures such as ice for treatment. A week later, the mass resolves, but she develops tender swelling in her left thigh with no known trauma to the area. The following lab studies are done.

CBC: WBC 11,300; normal differential; Hgb 10; Hct 30; MCV 78; Plts 202,000;
PT: 11.5 secs; PTT: 80 secs;
fibrinogen 350

The next appropriate studies for this patient's workup would be:

A. Lupus anticoagulant and anticardiolipin studies
B. 1:1 mix of patient and normal to measure the PTT
C. Repeat CBC
D. Platelet aggregation studies

308.

A 32-year-old woman presents with a mass under her tongue, followed by a thigh hematoma. She is otherwise healthy, but is noted to have a large spleen on exam.

Her laboratory studies are as follows:
CBC: WBC 110,300; 46% segs, 6% bands, 12% lymphs, 10% myelocytes, 8% metamyelocytes, 5% blasts, 7% eosinophils, 6% basophils, Hgb 10; Hct 30; MCV 85; Plts 898,000;
PT: 12 secs; PTT: 30 secs

Further workup for this patient should include:

A. Peripheral smear review, followed by bone marrow aspirate and cytogenetics
B. CT scan of the abdomen
C. FNA of the spleen
D. ANA

309.

A true statement concerning chronic lymphocytic leukemia (CLL) is:

A. Thrombocytopenia is diagnostic of stage 0 disease.
B. Thrombocytopenia is diagnostic of RAI stage III to IV disease.
C. Acquired von Willebrand disease with CLL is common.
D. AIHA and ITP are associated with CLL, but are always asymptomatic.

310.

A 36-year-old woman delivers her 3rd child and is discharged home in good health. The pregnancy and delivery were uncomplicated, and the infant is healthy. The mother returns within 48 hours complaining of abdominal pain and epistaxis. Her exam is benign with the exception of fresh blood in her posterior oropharynx.

Lab studies reveal the following:
    CBC: WBC 15,000; 75% segs, 10% bands, 15% lymphs; Hgb 8; Hct 24; Plts 4,000;
    PT: 12 secs; PTT: 32 secs;
    fibrinogen: 350

Her labs, when she was discharged, were completely normal. You review her current peripheral smear and note that her platelets are large, and she has many fragments and shift cells visible.

Appropriate further evaluation should include:

A. LDH, retic count, and antiplatelet antibody screen
B. LDH, retic count, and *ADAMTS13* testing
C. LDH, retic count, and Factor VIII level
D. LDH, retic count, and direct Coombs

311.

A 36-year-old woman delivers her 3rd child and is discharged home in good health. The pregnancy and delivery were uncomplicated, and the infant is healthy. The mother returns within 48 hours complaining of abdominal pain and epistaxis. Her exam is benign with the exception of fresh blood in her posterior oropharynx.

Lab studies reveal the following:
    CBC: WBC 15,000; 75% segs, 10% bands, 15% lymphs; Hgb 8; Hct 24; Plts 4,000;
    PT: 12 secs; PTT: 32 secs;
    fibrinogen: 350
    LDH 12,000; BUN 25; Retic count 5%; creatinine 3.5; total bili 5.0; Coombs negative; indirect bili 4.5;
    ALT 30; AST 35

Her labs, when she was discharged, were completely normal. You review her current peripheral smear and note that her platelets are large, and she has many fragments and shift cells visible.

You suspect this is pregnancy-associated thrombotic thrombocytopenic purpura (TTP).

Your next step in her management should be:

A. Placement of a catheter for therapeutic plasma exchange
B. Infusion of platelets
C. Infusion of FFP and platelets
D. Treatment with heparin

312.

A 34-year-old man presents with complaints of fatigue and weakness. He has noted a 10-pound weight loss over the last 3 weeks and some bruising on his legs. He feels as if he has a bad case of the flu. His wife was sick last week and is just now beginning to recover. You send him home with a prescription for oseltamivir (Tamiflu®). A week later, he returns with no improvement in his symptoms. Now he feels as if his gums are bleeding as well.

Lab studies reveal:
    CBC: WBC 110,000; 2% segs, 1% myelocytes, 97% blasts; Hgb 4; Hct 16; Plts 32,000;
    PT 12 scs; PTT 32 scs; fibrinogen 152

You review his peripheral smear and perform a bone marrow aspirate and biopsy with cytogenetics and flow cytometry. Your evaluation confirms this to be acute leukemia, more specifically AML.

The expected findings on the bone marrow aspirate with stains would be:

    A. Marrow fibrosis with no aspirate obtainable
    B. Sudan-positive cells
    C. PAS-positive cells
    D. Both PAS and TdT positivity of the marrow

313.

A 67-year-old female is admitted for acute cholecystitis.

    PMH: AVR secondary to bicuspid valve 6 months ago.
    Meds: warfarin, HCTZ, enalapril
    She is placed on a heparin infusion and transported to the OR for cholecystectomy, which is uneventful.
    On postoperative day 2, she develops a painful, swollen right lower extremity.
    CBC: WBC 12,500: 72% segs, 15% lymphs, 13% monos; Hgb 12.2, platelets 90,000
    D-dimer positive

Which of the following is the __most__ appropriate next step in patient care?

    A. Change heparin to LMWH.
    B. Discontinue heparin.
    C. Plasma exchange transfusion.
    D. Evaluate for *Factor V Leiden*, prothrombin gene mutation, and antiphospholipid antibodies.
    E. Fibrin split products.

314.

A 36-year-old female with a medical history of Hashimoto hypothyroidism and Ménière disease presents complaining of paresthesias in both big toes when wearing sandals. Exam reveals a gray forelock and scattered lymph nodes palpable to less than 1 centimeter in the anterior cervical region.

Neuro exam reveals normal sensation and proprioception. Lower-extremity vascular exam is normal.

    CBC: WBC 8,500 with normal differential
    Hgb 12.7, MCV 92, platelets 350,000
    Fasting blood glucose 82
    TSH 0.7 (0.5–5.0)
    Normal chemistry panel

Which of the following is the <u>most</u> appropriate next step in management?

    A. EMG and nerve conduction velocities
    B. MRI of the lumbar spine
    C. Test urine for heavy metals
    D. HbA1c testing
    E. B_{12}, folate, MMA, and homocysteine levels

315.

A 42-year-old woman with no complaints presents as a new patient after a recent move. Medical history includes iron deficiency anemia and hypothyroidism. She is adherent to her medications, including iron tid and levothyroxine.

Physical exam is normal.

    CBC: WBC 9,500 and normal differential
    Hgb 10.9, MCV 62, platelets 375,000
    Serum iron and ferritin normal
    CBC from 3 years previously: Hgb 10.1, MCV 65
    TSH 1.7 (0.5–5.0)

Which of the following is the <u>most</u> appropriate next step in patient care?

    A. Schedule a bone marrow biopsy.
    B. Order hemoglobin electrophoresis.
    C. Diagnose her with alpha thalassemia and discontinue supplemental iron.
    D. Transfuse with packed red cells.
    E. Order a Coombs test.

316.

An 82-year-old woman presents to her local emergency department with complaints of a mass under her tongue. Evaluation reveals it to be a large hematoma, and she is sent home with instructions to use local measures for treatment. A week later, the mass resolves, but she spontaneously develops a tender swelling in her left thigh. She has never had any bleeding problems in the past. She denies any history of easy bruising or bleeding gums.

CBC: WBC 11,300 and normal differential
Hgb 10, Hct 30, MCV 78, platelets 202,000
PT 11.5, PTT 80, Fibrinogen 350

Which of the following studies is <u>most</u> appropriate?

    A. Antiphospholipid antibodies
    B. 1:1 mix of patient's serum with control and measure PTT
    C. RIPA
    D. vWF:Ag, vWF:RCoF, and bleeding time
    E. Antiplatelet antibody

317.

A 19-year-old female with Hgb SC disease presents with complaints of abdominal pain. Medical history includes infrequent pain crises. Her current pain began acutely this evening after participating in a 5K walk for diabetes.

Exam: T 100° F, RR 12, BP 85/50, HR 110
Pallor and painful splenomegaly
WBC 14,500, 90% segs, 5% bands, 5% lymphs
Hgb 6.5 (normally 9.5), platelets 400,000
Retic count 7.9%

Which of the following is the <u>most</u> appropriate next step in patient care?

    A. Intravenous ceftriaxone and vancomycin
    B. Morphine, oxygen, and IV fluids
    C. Dopamine infusion
    D. Blood transfusion and surgical consultation
    E. Gall bladder ultrasound

318.

A 17-year-old female complains of episodes of RUQ pain x 2 weeks.

Gall bladder U/S = cholelithiasis
WBC 10,500 (normal differential)
Hgb 10.2, MCV 94
Platelets 400,000
Reticulocyte count 5.7%
Normal chemistries
AST 24, ALT 35, Alka phos 110
T. bili 4.5, D. bili 0.5, I. bili 4.0

Which of the following is the <u>most</u> likely associated laboratory finding?

A. Spherocytes on smear
B. Hypercholesterolemia
C. Hypertriglyceridemia
D. Teardrops on smear
E. Smudge cells on smear

319.

A 67-year-old female complains of rapidly growing neck swelling.

Weight loss of 15 lbs in 2 months
Exam = Multiple rubbery lymph nodes and palpable spleen
WBC 9,500 (70% segs, 15% eos, 10% lymphs, 5% monos)
Hgb 11.5 (MCV 90)
Platelets 350,000
Reticulocyte count 4.5%
T. Bili 3.7, I. Bili 3.2
AST 15, ALT 25
BUN 10, Creat 0.6

Which of the following is the <u>most</u> likely cause of the patient's anemia?

A. Iron deficiency
B. B_{12} deficiency
C. Chronic disease
D. Autoimmune hemolytic anemia
E. Acute leukemia

320.

An 18-year-old female complains of fatigue.

She has normal menses.
Exam is normal <u>except</u> for pallor.

    Hgb 10, MCV 70, Platelets 450,000
    Fe low, TIBC increased, ferritin low, % sat 10

She is given iron supplements.
At follow-up, she complains of persistent fatigue, abdominal fullness, and intermittent nausea. Bowel movements are "dark" and sometimes voluminous.

Repeat CBC shows a microcytic anemia that is unimproved.

Which of the following is the <u>most</u> appropriate next step in management?

    A. Coombs test.
    B. HIV ELISA.
    C. IgA tTGA.
    D. Emphasize a need for strict adherence to the iron supplements.
    E. Measurement of haptoglobin.

321.

The Philadelphia chromosome is found in which of the following disorders 95% of the time?

    A. CML
    B. CLL
    C. AML
    D. ALL

322.

A 54-year-old man with a history of prostate cancer postradical prostatectomy presents with complaints of fatigue and exertional pain in his back for 2 months. Exam shows normal straight leg raises, normal hip flexors, and down-going toes.

WBC 8,900 (normal differential)
Hgb 10.7
Hct 32
Platelets 310,000
Na 137
K 3.4
Cl 115
HCO_3 19
BUN 10, Creat 1.7
T. Prot 8.5, Alb 2.9
Ca 10.4
U/A: 2+ glucose, 2+ protein, no blood
Chest radiograph: Normal

Which of the following is <u>most</u> likely to diagnose <u>the cause</u> of his back pain?

A. Bone scan
B. Measurement of PSA
C. Serum and urine protein electrophoresis
D. Radiographs of the L-spine
E. MRI of the L-spine

323.

A 23-year-old male presents for evaluation of fatigue. He reports that he recently had a cold with upper respiratory cough, congestion, and malaise 2 weeks ago. His symptoms seemed to improve, but has noted worsening fatigue and malaise. He notes that he even feels short of breath when getting up to walk the last two days. His past medical history is significant for a cholecystectomy 7 years ago.

PE reveals a well-developed male with appropriate vital signs. He appears somewhat pale. He has a 1/6 faint systolic murmur at the lower left sternal border that does <u>not</u> radiate. Abdominal exam is notable for a palpable spleen tip.

CBC shows the following:
WBC 6.0
Hgb 7.5
Hct 22.3
Plt 190
MCV 78
MCHC 36

Which of the following would confirm the diagnosis?

A. Hemoglobin electrophoresis
B. G6PD enzyme activity
C. Osmotic fragility testing
D. Abdominal ultrasound
E. Serum LDH

324.

You are asked to consult on a 26-year-old female who was admitted to the trauma service following a motor vehicle accident. She experienced a fracture of the right femur that required internal fixation. Following surgery, the patient did well until this morning when she was noted to have right lower leg pain and swelling and chest pain with shortness of breath. She also developed marked weakness of the left arm and left leg. The patient is alert but in some distress.

The right-sided neurological findings are most likely related to:

A. Disseminated sepsis from a left leg cellulitis
B. Hypoxia from a pulmonary embolus
C. The presence of a persistent atrial septal defect
D. Unrecognized spinal cord trauma

325.

A 43-year-old man presents with polyuria. The patient has a paternal history of prostate cancer and is concerned about his symptoms. He has been having frequent urination for the last 2 months and urinating every 2 hours, day or night. He complains of fatigue, which interferes with his activity—he is an avid marathon runner and typically runs 1–2 marathons per year. He is currently able to run 5 miles before he becomes short of breath. His past medical, family, and social history are otherwise unremarkable.

His review of systems is significant for decreased sex drive and complaints of worsening hand pain over the last 3 months.

On physical exam, he is well tanned, fit, and in no distress. His heart and lung exam is normal. He has hepatomegaly on abdominal exam, without abdominal pain or masses. His exam is otherwise unremarkable.

Laboratory studies are significant for a hemoglobin A1c of 8.2%. A CBC is normal, as is a basic metabolic panel except for a glucose of 236 mg/dL.

What diagnostic tests should be ordered next?

A. Fasting lipid panel and urine microalbumin
B. Ferritin and transferrin
C. TSH, T_4 and T_3, and random cortisol level
D. PSA

326.

You see a 23-year-old male with a history of prolonged bleeding episodes and epistaxis for many years. He presented to the emergency department with a particularly difficult-to-control case of epistaxis. He has never had an evaluation for a bleeding disorder.

Laboratory results:
PT: normal
PTT: 55 seconds (control 34 seconds)
CBC: normal with normal platelets
Bleeding time: prolonged
Factor VII levels: normal
RIPA (platelet aggregation in response to ristocetin) is abnormal.

Which of the following is the most likely diagnosis?

A. Factor XIII deficiency
B. von Willebrand disease
C. Factor VII deficiency
D. Bernard-Soulier syndrome
E. Vitamin K deficiency

327.

A 70-year-old woman presents with complaints of spontaneous bruising on her forearms and thighs. You note large ecchymosis but no petechia or purpura on her exam. You order screening labs and find that her CBC is normal; however, her coagulations studies are not.

PT: 11 secs
PTT: 78 secs

You order mixing studies, which have the following results:
PTT: 78 secs
1:1 mix PTT: 32 secs
30-min incubation PTT: 40 secs
1-hour incubation PTT: 62 secs

These results can be best explained by which of the following?

A. She has a Factor X deficiency and must have an occult diagnosis of amyloid.
B. She most likely has a Factor VIII deficiency.
C. She most likely has a Factor IX deficiency.
D. She most likely has an inhibitor to Factor VIII.
E. She is taking warfarin.

328.

A 35-year-old woman is brought to the hospital by her friends for evaluation of change in mental status. She has had a fever and intermittent confusion for 3 days. Prior to this episode, she has been healthy.

Physical examination reveals a weak-appearing young woman with pallor. She is confused and is unable to give you any history. She has a temperature of 102° F. Her physical examination is normal except for the pallor and scattered petechiae.

Laboratory:
Hemoglobin: 9 mg/dL
Hematocrit: 35%
WBC: 6,700/mm^3 with a normal differential.
Platelets: 20,000
Peripheral smear shows many of the following:

Urinalysis shows numerous WBCs, RBCs, hemoglobin, and protein.
BUN: 47 mg/dL
Creatinine: 2.6 mg/dL
PT and PTT are normal.

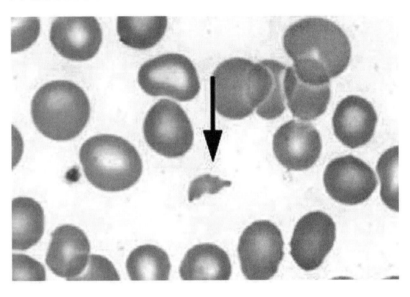

Which of the following is the most likely diagnosis?

A. DIC
B. Hemolytic uremic syndrome
C. Idiopathic thrombocytopenic purpura
D. Thrombotic thrombocytopenic purpura
E. Glanzmann thrombasthenia

329.

A 60-year-old man presents with weakness. His wife is there and says that he "drinks a lot."
You order laboratory and get a peripheral smear (see below).

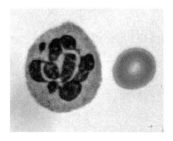

Based on the peripheral smear, which abnormality is <u>most</u> likely?

    A. Iron deficiency anemia
    B. Vitamin B_{12} deficiency
    C. ALL
    D. TTP
    E. ITP

330.

A patient with chronic uremia presents for evaluation. A peripheral smear is performed and shows the following:

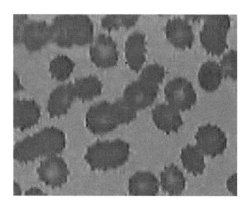

What is the abnormality seen on the peripheral smear?

    A. Iron deficiency anemia
    B. Burr cells (echinocytes)
    C. Schistocytes
    D. Histiocytes
    E. Target cells

331.

A 40-year-old woman presents for routine examination for life insurance credentialing. She is a nonsmoker and reports no family history of diseases, <u>except</u> that her mother had an "anemia," and she thinks one of her sisters may have it as well. She denies any health problems herself. Her insurance company requires lab and a peripheral smear:

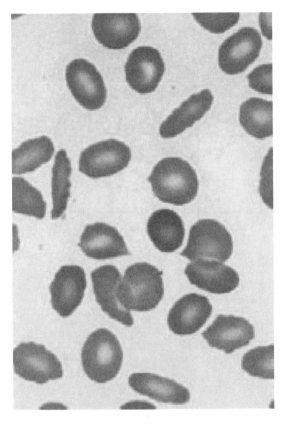

She is <u>not</u> anemic, but her reticulocyte count is elevated at 3.5%.

What is the <u>most</u> likely diagnosis?

    A. Asymptomatic vitamin B_{12} deficiency
    B. Hereditary pyropoikilocytosis
    C. Hereditary elliptocytosis
    D. Thalassemia trait
    E. Sickle cell disease

332.

Identify the abnormal cell in this peripheral smear:

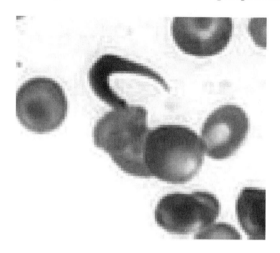

- A. Helmet cell
- B. Schistocyte
- C. Plasma cell
- D. Sickle cell
- E. Elliptocyte

333.

Examine the following cell seen in a peripheral smear.

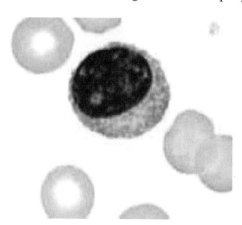

Which of the following diseases is this cell associated with?

- A. Multiple myeloma.
- B. Waldenström macroglobulinemia.
- C. MGUS (Monoclonal gammopathy of uncertain significance).
- D. Plasma cell leukemia.
- E. All of the options are associated with this type of cell.

334.

Examine the following peripheral smear and identify the abnormal cell designated by the arrow.

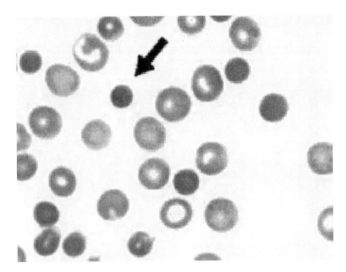

    A. Sickle cell
    B. Elliptocyte
    C. Plasma cell
    D. Helmet cell
    E. Spherocyte

335.

Examine the following peripheral smear:

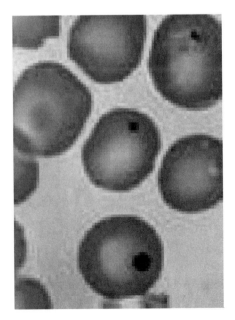

Which of the following has <u>most</u> likely occurred in this patient?

   A. Liver biopsy
   B. Blood transfusion
   C. Splenectomy
   D. Cholecystectomy

336.

Examine the following peripheral smear:

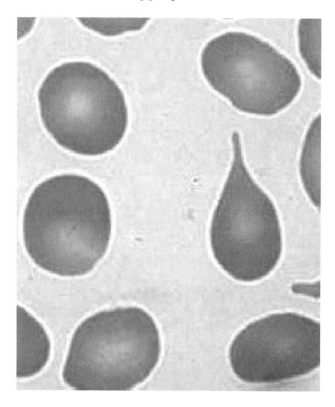

What disease process is associated with this peripheral smear?

   A. Thalassemia
   B. Sickle cell anemia
   C. ALL
   D. Microangiopathic hemolytic anemia
   E. Sideroblastic anemia

337.

A 24-year-old with known sickle cell disease presents to the emergency room complaining of extreme fatigue and shortness of breath. Laboratory testing reveals: hemoglobin: 4.4 g/dL, hematocrit: 12.5%, and reticulocyte count: 0.2%. PT and PTT are normal.

What is the <u>most</u> likely cause of his symptoms?

    A. Parvovirus B19 infection
    B. *Salmonella* septicemia
    C. Pneumococcal septicemia
    D. Cerebrovascular occlusion with hemorrhagic stroke
    E. Pulmonary infarction with acute chest syndrome

338.

A 39-year-old man presents with a history of hepatomegaly and high red blood count without apparent cause. He has been well until earlier today when he developed sudden onset of pain in his right upper quadrant.

On examination:

    Afebrile, BP 135/88, P 110, RR 18

HEENT:	WNL
Heart:	RRR without murmurs, rubs, or gallops
Lungs:	CTA
Abdomen:	Markedly enlarged liver that is very tender on its edge.
	Spleen is enlarged.
	A fluid wave is present.

Laboratory:
    CBC is pending, but his last known hemoglobin was 18 mg/dL.
    AST is 110.
    ALT is 86.

A Doppler study was nondiagnostic.

What is the next procedure you should consider?

    A. MRI angiography or hepatic venography
    B. HIDA scan
    C. Paracentesis
    D. Radionucleotide liver-spleen scan

339.

A 47-year-old man with Zollinger-Ellison syndrome presents with a 3-month history of anemia. Physical exam is unremarkable.

Medications: Hydrochlorothiazide, sildenafil, sertraline, omeprazole, and diphenhydramine
Lab: Hb 10.5 mg/dL, Hct 30%, MCV 114, WBC 3.6

What is the <u>most</u> likely cause for his anemia?

    A. Lead toxicity
    B. Alcohol
    C. Folate deficiency
    D. B_{12} deficiency
    E. Sideroblastic anemia

ONCOLOGY

340.

A 64-year-old smoker arrives at your office with complaints of abdominal pain and constipation, worsening over the last 2 months. He has never experienced anything like this before. He has a chronic nonproductive cough and a 10-pound weight loss but is otherwise healthy. His physical exam is unremarkable.

Lab studies include: CBC: WBC 4,200, normal differential, Hgb 12, Hct 36, MCV 86, Plts 250,000

Chemistries: Na 136   Cl 108   Bun 10
            K 4.0 HCO_3 24   Creat 2.2
            Mg 1.8   Ca 12.0   Alb 2.0

Initial treatment for his complaints should include:

A. IV normal saline for hydration
B. pRBCs for anemia
C. Laxative for constipation
D. Treatment for probable IBS

341.

A 65-year-old man with long history of smoking and solitary pulmonary nodule presents with hypercalcemia.

Which of the following cancers is <u>most</u> likely?

A. Metastatic prostate cancer
B. Large cell lung cancer
C. Metastatic testicular cancer
D. Squamous cell lung cancer

342.

A 25-year-old male presents with painless swelling of his scrotum for 2 months. The swelling is worsening and has begun to worry him. He is otherwise healthy. His physical exam confirms scrotal swelling with testicular enlargement.

Initial work up should be:

A. MRI head
B. CT abdomen
C. Ultrasound of testicle
D. Laparoscopic removal of the testicle

343.

A 19-year-old man presents with a 2-month history of having a testicular mass. An ultrasound is done and reveals a solid mass. Testicular cancer is suspected.

The next step should be:

A. AFP, BHCG, transscrotal removal of the testicle
B. CEA, LDH, transscrotal removal of the testicle
C. AFP, BHCG, inguinal orchiectomy
D. CEA, LDH, inguinal orchiectomy

344.

A 21-year-old male with a testicular mass undergoes inguinal orchiectomy. His lab returns, and his chemistries are normal, as is his CBC. Other values include:

LDH 1,000, BHCG 0, AFP 2,000, CEA 0

His pathologic diagnosis is a testicular seminoma.

You should now:

A. Begin treatment for a nonseminoma.
B. Begin treatment for a seminoma.
C. Have the pathology reviewed.
D. Remove the remaining testicle prophylactically.

345.

A 52-year-old woman presents after finding a small mass in her left breast on self-examination. She has no family history of malignancy, and she has never had a mammogram.

You should now:

A. Offer her reassurance that a negative family history is protective.
B. Offer her lumpectomy to remove the mass.
C. Watch the mass with serial exams for 3–6 months.
D. Send her for a mammogram and possible ultrasound of the mass.

346.

A 52-year-old woman presents after finding a small mass in her left breast on self-examination. She has no family history of malignancy, and she has never had a mammogram. You recommend that she undergo mammogram and undergo ultrasound of the mass. She failed to keep her scheduled follow-up and returns to see you a year later. Now the mass is 6 cm, firm, and fixed to her chest wall; she has matted nodes in her axilla. FNA of the mass is read as intraductal carcinoma.

Treatment options include:

A. Modified radical mastectomy with axillary node dissection
B. Lumpectomy and axillary node dissection
C. Lumpectomy with axillary node dissection and axillary radiation therapy
D. Neoadjuvant radiation therapy, followed by appropriate surgery

---

347.

A woman with a breast mass and axillary nodal disease has a modified radical mastectomy with axillary node dissection. Pathology confirms intraductal carcinoma with 8/10 positive lymph nodes and negative staining: HER2/neu, ER, PR.

She should now receive:

A. Adjuvant hormonal treatment with tamoxifen or an aromatase inhibitor
B. Adjuvant chemotherapy with a combination of drugs
C. No further treatment because her disease has been completely resected
D. Chemotherapy followed by tamoxifen or an aromatase inhibitor

---

348.

A 52-year-old woman has intraductal carcinoma with 8/10 lymph nodes positive on axillary dissection. She is HER2/neu, ER, and PR negative for all. She is the first woman in the family to have breast cancer that any relatives can remember.

Current screening recommendations would now indicate her female family members should:

A. Be tested for *BRCA1* and *BRCA2*.
B. Have mammograms starting at age 20 and yearly thereafter.
C. Follow routine screening evaluation as appropriate for their age.
D. Have yearly mammograms and ultrasounds starting at age 50.

349.

Many neoplastic lesions are recognizably abnormal by microscopy but are so similar to each other that differentiating them is a pathologist's challenge. This process is assisted by a multitude of stains and cellular markers that allow different tumors to be identified by their specific pattern of response. For example, desmin is very useful in distinguishing small cell tumors that are otherwise very similar to each other.

Which type of small cell tumor would be expected to test positive for the tumor marker desmin?

A. Alveolar rhabdomyosarcoma
B. Neuroblastoma
C. Lymphoma
D. Soft tissue Ewing sarcoma
E. Undifferentiated small cell carcinoma

350.

A 37-year-old female comes to your clinic to request breast cancer screening. Her 46-year-old sister was recently diagnosed with bilateral breast cancer. Your patient is anxious to pursue active surveillance and specifically requests gene testing to evaluate her breast cancer risk.

Which of the following statements regarding this testing is <u>most</u> accurate?

    A. The majority of breast cancer cases are associated with *BRCA* mutations.
    B. *BRCA* analysis is recommended as a general adjunct to mammography.
    C. Individuals with *BRCA* mutations benefit from preventive chemotherapy.
    D. Maternal ovarian cancer at age 37 years is an indication for *BRCA* testing.

351.

A 67-year-old female who presented with rectal bleeding undergoes diagnostic colonoscopy. A 2.5-cm tumor was noted in the mid-descending colon, and biopsy results revealed the diagnosis of adenocarcinoma.

Of the following, which intervention is <u>most</u> likely to result in cure?

    A. Radiation therapy
    B. Surgical excision
    C. Chemotherapy
    D. Immunotherapy

352.

You see a 36-year-old woman for persistent cough and increasing shortness of breath over the past 6 weeks. She was evaluated in an urgent care center 4 weeks ago, given the diagnosis of bronchitis, and placed on doxycycline. Her symptoms did <u>not</u> resolve, and 2 weeks ago the physician at the urgent care center ordered a chest x-ray. Based on the x-ray, the patient was told she had pneumonia, and the physician called in a 5-day course of azithromycin. Since then, she continues to cough up a large amount of watery sputum with occasional blood and "flecks of tissue." For a week now, she has demonstrable shortness of breath with exertion and low-grade fevers but no rigors. She has no significant medical history, does <u>not</u> drink alcohol or smoke cigarettes, and has never used illicit drugs. Her only medications are over-the-counter cough medicine and acetaminophen for fevers. Review of systems is remarkable for a 12-pound weight loss over the course of the last few months and night sweats for the past 3 weeks.

On physical exam, she appears acutely ill, thin, but well nourished.

Vital signs: BP 110/70 mmHg, P 90, R 22, T 38.5° C (101.3° F)

HEENT, cardiovascular, abdominal, and neurologic exams are normal.

Lung exam is positive for diffuse rhonchi, crackles at the bases, and egophony throughout the lung fields. Oxygen saturation on room air is 93%.

WBC is 8,200 cells/mm^3, with differential: 68 neutrophils, 3 bands, 8 eosinophils, 21 lymphocytes.

Chest x-ray shows diffuse, bilateral fluffy infiltrates throughout all lung fields and air bronchograms, with small bilateral pleural effusions.

Which of the following is the _most_ likely diagnosis?

A. Idiopathic pulmonary fibrosis
B. Congestive heart failure
C. Bronchoalveolar carcinoma
D. *Pneumocystis jiroveci* (formerly *Pneumocystis carinii*) pneumonia
E. Chronic eosinophilic pneumonitis

353.

Your patient is a 23-year-old female with a history of Hodgkin lymphoma diagnosed at age 21 years. During her treatment for this disease, she received chemotherapy, including doxorubicin, bleomycin, vincristine, and dacarbazine. She presents to clinic at this time with complaints of shortness of breath and a persistent dry, hacking cough.

Which of the following chemotherapeutic agents is _most_ likely to be related to her current complaints?

A. Doxorubicin
B. Bleomycin
C. Vincristine
D. Dacarbazine

354.

A 40-year-old man presents to the clinic with a "lump" in his groin. He has noticed some lower abdominal pain associated with the lump, but has no other PMH or symptoms. He is overweight, but takes no medications, uses no tobacco, and admits to modest alcohol consumption. There is no significant family history. ROS is otherwise negative.

The exam is normal with the exception of a left-sided varicocele, which persists when the patient is recumbent.

Labs results:

Na:	138 mEq/dL
Cl:	102 mEq/dL
K:	3.8 mEq/dL
HCO$_3$:	26 mEq/dL
BUN:	32 mg/dL
Cr:	1.3 mg/dL
Glu:	116 mg/dL
WBC:	8.5 cells/mm^3
Hb:	18.0 g/dL
Hct:	53.5%
Plt:	274,000 cells/mm^3

U/A: 1.024, 5.0, 2 WBCs, 5 RBCs, 1+ blood; otherwise negative.

Which of the following is the <u>most</u> appropriate next step in patient care?

    A. Referral to a urologist for semi-urgent repair of the varicocele.
    B. Referral to hematology for phlebotomy and bone marrow biopsy.
    C. Urine cytology, abdominal CT to rule out an abdominal malignancy.
    D. Send serum markers for testicular carcinoma (AFP, beta-HCG); perform testicular ultrasound.
    E. Referral for fertility counseling.

355.

A 62-year-old female returns for follow-up after consultation with the local gastroenterologist, where an upper endoscopic procedure with biopsies was performed. Review of the pathology report reveals the presence of extranodal marginal zone B lymphoma of MALT type in the gastric mucosa. As you discuss the treatment options with the patient, you mention the possibility that toxic chemotherapeutic agents may <u>not</u> be required due to the frequent cause of this disease.

The etiologic agent associated with this process is:

    A. Epstein-Barr virus (EBV)
    B. *Helicobacter pylori* (*H. pylori*)
    C. Hepatitis B virus
    D. Human herpesvirus 8
    E. *Tropheryma whipplei*

356.

A 27-year-old female presents to clinic for pelvic examination and Pap smear. She has had *Chlamydia* twice in the past and *Trichomonas* once in the previous 9 years. Her last Pap smear was two years ago, and she has missed two scheduled follow-ups. She reports previous abnormalities with her Pap smears but does <u>not</u> know the results. She has no acute complaints.

On pelvic examination, external genitalia are unremarkable. There is no discharge. Cervical DNA probes and a wet mount are obtained. Pap specimen is obtained without difficulty, and no lesions are visualized. Bimanual examination reveals no abnormalities.

The DNA probes are negative for *Chlamydia* and gonorrhea. Wet mount is normal. Pap results indicated adequate specimen, and pathology is reported as atypical squamous cells of undetermined significance (ASCUS). Reflex human papilloma virus (HPV) studies are positive for a high-risk subtype of papilloma virus.

Which of the following is <u>most</u> appropriate for this patient?

    A. Repeat Pap smear in one year.
    B. Repeat Pap smear in 3–6 months.
    C. Colposcopy.
    D. Acetic acid applications.
    E. Podophyllin application to the cervix.

357.

A 52-year-old, long-term male patient of your practice presents with complaints of left knee pain and swelling, which has been progressing over the last 3–4 weeks. He is <u>not</u> aware of any trauma or injury. His past history is most remarkable for blindness secondary to bilateral enucleation. He was diagnosed at age 18 months with a retinoblastoma in the left eye. At 24 months, a second tumor was noted in the right eye. He is also on hydrochlorothiazide for treatment of essential hypertension and a statin for hyperlipidemia.

On x-ray, the patient is noted to have a lytic disruption in the metaphyseal region of the proximal left tibia.

Which of the following is the <u>most</u> likely diagnosis?

   A. Osteogenic sarcoma
   B. Ewing sarcoma
   C. Multiple myeloma
   D. Parathyroid tumors

358.

A 24-year-old male with a known history of HIV presents with scattered peripheral lymphadenopathy. He is referred for biopsy, and the pathologist reports Burkitt lymphoma. In consultation with oncology, the patient is admitted for staging and initiation of therapy. On the second day of treatment, you are called by nursing, who reports a marked decrease in urine output.

Laboratory results:

	Admission	Current	Normals
Sodium:	141	138	135–146 mmol/L
Potassium:	4.5	6.4	3.5–5.3 mmol/L
Chloride:	108	101	98–110 mmol/L
Bicarbonate:	27	21	21–33 mmol/L
Calcium:	8.9	7.1	8.5–10.4 mg/dL
Phosphate:	3.6	8.2	2.5–4.5 mg/dL
Uric acid:	7.6	12.2	2.5–8.0 mg/dL
BUN:	14	42	7–25 mg/dL
Creatinine:	1.1	1.9	0.5–1.2 mg/dL

Early treatment with which of the following would <u>most</u> likely have prevented this patient's condition?

   A. Therapy with intravenous steroids
   B. Pretreatment with oral allopurinol
   C. Intravenous infusion of calcium
   D. Acidification of the urine

359.

A 26-year-old male graduate student is seen in a campus health clinic with concerns regarding a lump he has found in his right testicle. It is <u>not</u> painful. He is sexually active with his wife of 4 years. Past history is remarkable for surgical correction of an undescended right testicle at 2 years of age; tonsillectomy at age 6, secondary to recurrent childhood infections; and appendectomy at age 16.

On physical examination, there is fullness and an eccentric mass on the lateral aspect of his right testicle. He complains of mild tenderness on palpation. The lesion does <u>not</u> transilluminate. Exam of the left testicle is unremarkable.

Which of the following is the <u>most</u> likely diagnosis?

   A. Varicocele
   B. Spermatocele
   C. Hydrocele
   D. Germ cell tumor

360.

You are asked to meet with a 64-year-old male and his family. He was recently diagnosed with non-Hodgkin lymphoma, and the family is seeking information regarding the prognosis for this patient.

In reviewing his case, which of the following prognostic indicators for non-Hodgkin lymphoma is associated with the best outcome?

   A. Age older than 60
   B. Lymph node involvement of the spleen, splenic hilar nodes, and celiac nodes only
   C. Pathology diagnostic of diffuse large B-cell lymphoma
   D. Neoplastic cells noted on bone marrow aspiration but without other recognized sites
   E. Lymph node involvement limited to mediastinum and abdominal para-aortic nodes

---

361.

A 60-year-old man is referred to you for weight loss. He says he has lost 40 pounds in the past 3 months without dieting. He describes feeling full after only a few bites of food. He has also noted some abdominal fullness and swelling over the last 2 weeks and that his ankles have been swelling for the last few days. He denies any other complaints and has no chronic medical problems.

On physical exam, he has a large abdominal mass that is firm and nontender. There is no lymphadenopathy, and the rest of his exam is normal. You refer him to a general surgeon, and biopsy of the mass is consistent with a diagnosis of Burkitt lymphoma.

Which of the treatment regimens is associated with Burkitt lymphoma?

   A. This is a common subtype of NHL, and treatment is hormonal.
   B. This is an indolent lymphoma and requires no immediate treatment.
   C. This is a very aggressive lymphoma that does not respond to treatment.
   D. Treatment should include CNS prophylaxis.

362.

A 42-year-old man presents with fatigue and weight loss. He also notes that he has had a "knot" in his leg for the last month, which seems to be enlarging. He has had no chronic health issues and has <u>not</u> seen a doctor since childhood. His physical exam is unremarkable <u>except</u> for a 6-cm mass in his left thigh.

Laboratory results:
Hemoglobin:	8 g/dL
WBC:	800,230 cells/mm^3
Segmented neutrophils:	30%
Bands:	10%
Lymphs:	7%
Blasts:	20%
Myelocytes:	22%
Basophils:	8%
Eosinophils:	3%
Hematocrit:	25%
Platelets:	130,000 cells/mm^3

He is admitted to the hospital for continued evaluation.

Which of the following is the <u>most</u> appropriate next step in patient care?

    A. A bleeding time followed by biopsy of the thigh mass
    B. A LAP (leukocyte alkaline phosphatase)
    C. Bone marrow aspirate and biopsy
    D. Emergent leukophoresis
    E. Peripheral blood flow cytometry and cytogenetics

363.

A 50-year-old male smoker presents for evaluation at the request of his wife. He had been previously healthy but developed a cough with two episodes of self-limited hemoptysis two months ago. Medical history is significant for hypertension and hyperlipidemia. He does <u>not</u> use drugs or alcohol. He earned his living as a stockbroker and is now retired. Review of systems is positive for 15-pound weight loss in spite of a normal appetite, 3x/night nocturia, and excessive thirst.

Medications: HCTZ 25 QD, atorvastatin 10 mg QHS
PE: Normal vital signs.
Head and neck is normal.

Lungs show symmetric expansion, resonance to percussion, vesicular breath sounds throughout with occasional expiratory wheezes and course crackles on the left.

Screening laboratories reveal:
Hgb:	10.2 g/dL
Platelets:	180,000 cells/mm^3
Na:	137 mEq/L
K:	3.8 mEq/L
Cl:	92 mEq/L

HCO₃: 23 mEq/L
BUN: 8 mg/dL
Creatinine: 0.8 mg/dL
Glucose: 110 mg/dL
Calcium: 10.8 mg/dL
Albumin: 2.0 g/dL

Chest radiograph shows a central lung mass measuring 3 cm.

Which of the following is the <u>most</u> likely diagnosis?

    A. Small cell lung cancer
    B. Adenocarcinoma
    C. Squamous cell lung cancer
    D. Large cell lung cancer

364.

A 64-year-old previously healthy man presents for evaluation of cough. Two months ago, he developed a cough that has become chronic and nonproductive. In the last two weeks, he began having a sensation of "fullness in the left side of my chest." This has worsened, resulting in his scheduling his appointment. He takes no medicines and has no medical history. He does <u>not</u> smoke cigarettes or use drugs or alcohol. He is a police officer and has <u>not</u> traveled outside of his hometown of Galveston, Texas, in the past 5 years. Review of systems is positive only for fatigue. He specifically denies fevers.

PE: Normal vital signs.
Head and neck is normal.

Lungs show symmetric expansion, resonance on the right and decreased resonance to percussion in the left mid-lung zone, vesicular breath sounds throughout with occasional expiratory wheezes, and coarse crackles on the left.

Screening laboratories reveal:
    Hgb: 10.2 g/dL
    Platelets: 180,000 cells/mm³
    Na: 137 mEq/L
    K: 3.8 mEq/L
    Cl: 92 mEq/L
    HCO₃: 23 mEq/L
    BUN: 8 mg/dL
    Creatinine: 0.8 mg/dL
    Glucose: 110 mg/dL
    Calcium: 8.8 mg/dL
    Albumin: 2.0 g/dL

Chest radiograph reveals a consolidated left middle lobe.

Which of the following is the <u>most</u> likely diagnosis?

    A. Small cell lung cancer
    B. Bronchoalveolar cancer (BAC)
    C. Squamous cell lung cancer
    D. Community-acquired pneumonia (CAP)
    E. Metastatic melanoma

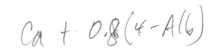

$$Ca + 0.8(4 - Alb)$$

365.

A 55-year-old man presents for evaluation. He was previously healthy, but developed a cough two months ago; the cough was initially nonproductive, but over the past one month, the patient has experienced two episodes of self-limited hemoptysis. He has also lost 15 pounds in spite of a normal appetite. He takes no medicines and has no medical history. He has smoked 1 pack of cigarettes per day for the past 25 years; he does <u>not</u> use drugs or alcohol. In the past year, he has traveled to Oklahoma and Galveston. He does <u>not</u> hunt or go hiking in the woods. Review of systems is positive only for fatigue. He specifically denies fevers.

PE: Normal vital signs.
Head and neck is normal.

Lungs show symmetric expansion, resonance to percussion, vesicular breath sounds throughout with occasional expiratory wheezes and coarse crackles on the left.

Screening laboratories reveal:
Hgb:	10.2 g/dL
Platelets:	180,000 cells/mm^3
Na:	137 mEq/L
K:	3.8 mEq/L
Cl:	92 mEq/L
HCO$_3$:	23 mEq/L
BUN:	8 mg/dL
Creatinine:	0.8 mg/dL
Glucose:	110 mg/dL
Calcium:	8.8 mg/dL
Albumin:	2.0 g/dL

Chest radiograph reveals a central, cavitating tumor in his left lung.

Which of the following is the <u>most</u> likely diagnosis?

    A. Squamous cell lung cancer
    B. Adenocarcinoma
    C. Small cell lung cancer
    D. Large cell lung cancer
    E. Blastomycosis

366.

You see a 57-year-old woman in your office for fatigue and back pain. She has a history of hypertension, peptic ulcer disease, and breast cancer—for which she had a modified radical mastectomy and subsequent chemotherapy in 1998. She has been disease-free since then. In 2002, she was in a motor vehicle accident and states she has had lower back pain since. She usually performs back stretches twice a week.

She describes the pain as dull but worsening over the past five weeks. The pain is worse when she lies in bed. Her legs feel weak, and she is fatigued. There has been no weight loss.

There is no other medical history.

She takes HCTZ and omeprazole. She has no allergies.

Neurologic exam is significant for 4/5 power in the legs bilaterally, 3+ patellar and ankle reflexes, and uncoordinated gait. Straight-leg raises cause bilateral back pain with some radiation down the legs.

Pulses are 2+ and equal bilaterally.

Which of the following is the <u>most</u> appropriate next step in the management of this patient?

    A. X-rays of the spine
    B. Referral to orthopaedics for elective surgical evaluation
    C. Neurologic consultation, electromyelogram
    D. Dexamethasone intravenously, emergent spine MRI
    E. Physical therapy for lumbar spinal stenosis

367.

Your patient is a 33-year-old female with a history of lymphoma, which was diagnosed 3 months ago. During her treatment for this disease, she has been receiving chemotherapy, including doxorubicin, bleomycin, vincristine, and dacarbazine. She presents to clinic at this time with complaints of peripheral neuropathy.

Which of the following chemotherapeutic agents is <u>most</u> likely to be related to her current symptoms?

    A. Doxorubicin
    B. Bleomycin
    C. Vincristine
    D. Dacarbazine

368.

You have followed a patient for 3 years since her radiation treatment for Hodgkin disease. She received an upper mantle port for an apparent cure of her disease. At the time of her visit today, she complains of fatigue, hair loss, and weight gain.

Which of the following diagnostic tests is <u>most</u> appropriate in this person's evaluation?

A. Repeat CT scans of her chest and abdomen for disease assessment.
B. Chemistry panel showing calcium level.
C. TSH.
D. Pulmonary function tests.

369.

Which of the following is associated with this finding in a bone marrow aspirate with peroxidase staining?

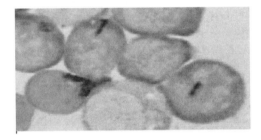

A. Acute lymphocytic leukemia (ALL)
B. Acute myelogenous leukemia (AML)
C. Chronic lymphocytic leukemia (CLL)
D. Chronic myelogenous leukemia (CML)
E. Hodgkin disease

370.

Which of the following chemotherapeutic agents is <u>most</u> commonly associated with renal toxicity?

A. Doxorubicin
B. Methotrexate
C. Vincristine
D. Vinblastine
E. Cisplatin

371.

A 50-year-old female presents to the clinic with complaints of perimenopausal symptoms. She experiences significant hot flashes, mood swings, and vaginal dryness. She has read about the adverse effects of hormone replacement, but is very interested in a course of tapering hormone replacement, specifically estrogen. She has never had any gynecologic surgeries.

If estrogen was given unopposed to this woman as part of a regimen provided to relieve her menopausal symptoms, for which of the following conditions would this patient be <u>most</u> at risk?

A. Breast cancer
B. Thromboembolic events
C. Cardiac disease
D. Endometrial cancer

372.

A 70-year-old man presents for evaluation at the request of his wife. He has been previously healthy but developed a cough two months ago; the cough was initially nonproductive, but over the past one month, the patient has experienced two episodes of self-limited hemoptysis. He has also lost 15 pounds in spite of a normal appetite. He takes no medicines and has no medical history. He smokes 1 pack of cigarettes per day and has done so for 35 years. He does <u>not</u> use drugs or alcohol.

PE: Normal vital signs.
Head and neck is normal.

Lungs show symmetric expansion, resonance to percussion, vesicular breath sounds throughout with occasional expiratory wheezes, and coarse crackles on the left.

Screening laboratories reveal:
Hgb:	10.2 g/dL
Platelets:	180,000 cells/mm^3
Na:	125 mEq/L
K:	3.8 mEq/L
Cl:	92 mEq/L
HCO$_3$:	23 mEq/L
BUN:	8 mg/dL
Creatinine:	0.8 mg/dL
Glucose:	110 mg/dL
Serum osm:	267 mOsm/kg

Chest radiograph shows a central lung mass measuring 3 cm.

Which of the following is the <u>most</u> likely diagnosis?

A. Small cell lung cancer
B. Adenocarcinoma
C. Squamous cell lung cancer
D. Large cell lung cancer
E. Blastomycosis

373.

A 23-year-old man presents with progressively worsening pain in the mid to proximal area of the left femur. It has awakened him each night over the past week. Acetaminophen and ibuprofen have offered no relief. He did try some aspirin the evening prior to presentation and noted some relief in the pain. He is clearly uncomfortable during the examination, which is significant for decreased strength in the left lower extremity. X-ray shows a round metaphyseal lucency surrounded by sclerotic bone.

Which of the following is the <u>most</u> likely diagnosis?

    A. Osteochondroma
    B. Ewing sarcoma
    C. Osteosarcoma
    D. Osteoid osteoma
    E. Fibrous dysplasia

374.

An 18-year-old college student has had poorly controlled atopic disease and recurrent infections associated with poor growth throughout his life. At birth, he had prolonged bleeding following circumcision. Workup at that time revealed thrombocytopenia, and he was diagnosed with Wiskott-Aldrich syndrome.

Of the following tumors, which should you be <u>most</u> vigilant about detecting during early adulthood?

    A. Renal cell carcinoma
    B. Malignant melanoma
    C. Lymphoma and leukemia
    D. Hepatic carcinoma
    E. Testicular seminoma

NEUROLOGY

375.

Which of the following factors predicts a better prognosis in people who have multiple sclerosis?

A. Male
B. Older age of onset
C. Many attacks within the first 2 years of the disease onset
D. Early in the course of the illness, having high disability
E. Few lesions on MRI

376.

A 34-year-old man is being treated for his partial seizure disorder (he has simple partial and complex partial seizures due to a past head injury) with carbamazepine.

Which of the following medications might decrease the serum concentration of carbamazepine?

A. Phenobarbital
B. Valproate
C. Lamotrigine
D. Levetiracetam
E. Gabapentin

377.

A 34-year-old woman is being treated for her partial seizure disorder (she has simple partial and complex partial seizures due to a past head injury) with carbamazepine. She is now considering becoming pregnant.

Which antiseizure medication would be an appropriate choice in order to maintain seizure control through her pregnancy?

A. Phenobarbital.
B. Valproate.
C. Lamotrigine.
D. Phenytoin.
E. None of these—stop her medications.

378.

A 30-year-old man has a sudden severe headache. He thinks that when the headache started, that he may have "passed out" for a "second." Upon arrival in the emergency department, he has neck stiffness, photophobia, and a blood pressure of 170/96. His exam is normal otherwise. CT scan shows blood in the suprasellar cistern and left sylvian fissure.

What is the next <u>most</u> appropriate test?

A. MRI brain.
B. Carotid Doppler.
C. Lumbar puncture.
D. Call neurosurgery!
E. 4-vessel angiography.

379.

A 70-year-old comes to the office with his wife. He has been having problems walking for about 2 years, and starting about 6 months ago, has been having increasing difficulty with short-term memory. On further questioning, it seems that he has also had several episodes of urinary incontinence over the past 1 year. On exam, his gait has a "magnetic" quality. He scores 27/30 on mini-mental status exam, missing 2/3 items on recall, and <u>not</u> recalling today's date. His MRI shows enlarged ventricles, with transependymal flow.

What is the <u>most</u> likely diagnosis?

A. Alzheimer's
B. Parkinson disease
C. Normal pressure hydrocephalus
D. Creutzfeldt-Jakob Disease

380.

A 55-year-old woman has frequent sinus infections and has been taking azithromycin for the past 10 days for a recurrence of this. However, during the past week, she has had headaches and has developed right-sided proptosis and double vision. On exam, there is decreased movement of the right eye and diminished sensation over the right forehead and cheek (normal over the right chin).

What is the cause of her neurological findings?

A. Cavernous sinus thrombosis
B. Sagittal sinus thrombosis
C. Right posterior communicating artery aneurysm
D. Left middle cerebral artery stroke
E. Ramsay-Hunt syndrome

381.

A 70-year-old who has hypertension, hyperlipidemia, and diabetes, all of which is poorly controlled, comes to the emergency department with acute onset of left leg weakness. The patient's daughter first noticed this, and the patient seems to be relatively unconcerned about this. On exam, you find weakness of the arm as well, but less obvious than the leg. There is no fever, chills, or recent illness.

Where is the <u>most</u> likely location of the stroke?

    A. Left anterior cerebral artery
    B. Right anterior cerebral artery
    C. Left middle cerebral artery
    D. Right middle cerebral artery

382.

A 47-year-old man is brought into the emergency department by his family because they thought they saw a seizure. When they first found him, he was lying on the couch, "shaking a little," and unresponsive. To the wife, he initially appeared "blue" around the lips. As he began to wake up, the family noticed right-sided weakness and "confusion" and called 911.

On arrival to the emergency department, he is afebrile. There is no neck stiffness. The patient is confused, but is following simple commands. When he talks, there is great hesitancy. However, he can repeat short phrases. He has mild weakness of the right face and arm. There is weakness of the right leg as well, but much less noticeable than the face.

He has no risk factors for heart disease (no hypertension, nonsmoker, no family history of heart disease). For several months, the family had noticed some word-finding problems, but they had joked that the patient was having "senile moments." He has been well, denied feeling sick, and has had no sick contacts.

What is the <u>most</u> likely diagnosis?

    A. Cerebral abscess
    B. Cerebral tumor
    C. Stroke
    D. Herpes encephalitis

383.

A 45-year-old man comes to his doctor's office with lower back pain. The pain started suddenly after he was lifting a couch as he and his wife were redecorating their living room. The pain radiates down the posterior right thigh to his right ankle. It is worse when he moves. On examination, he has difficulty performing strength testing because he is in pain (it hurts when he moves). The pain is brought out with right straight leg raises. He has a diminished right ankle jerk reflex.

What is the <u>most</u> likely diagnosis?

    A. Right L3–4 radiculopathy
    B. Right L4–5 radiculopathy
    C. Right L5–S1 radiculopathy
    D. Left L4–5 radiculopathy

384.

A 56-year-old man presents for routine follow-up and complains of one month of increasing stiffness and trouble getting started walking. ROS is otherwise negative.

Medical history includes DM, HTN, and newly diagnosed AIDS, which was diagnosed after an episode of psychosis 3 months ago.

Meds: AZT/3TC, efavirenz, reserpine, glipizide, HCTZ

Exam: Normal except for bilateral axillary lymphadenopathy, which is improving. No increased motor tone or rigidity. No tremor. Gait is slightly wide-based, and he has trouble starting from a stopped position. Cerebellar exam is normal.

Which of the following is the most appropriate next step in management?

   A. Start carbidopa/levodopa.
   B. Lumbar puncture and send CSF for JC virus PCR.
   C. Change efavirenz to nevirapine.
   D. Discontinue reserpine.
   E. Referral to a neurologist.

385.

A 26-year-old female attorney has a severe, retro-orbital, stabbing headache for twenty minutes. It awakens her from sleep each morning at 2 a.m. and has done so for the past 5 days. She has no prior history of headache. Medical history and family history are negative. She attended a wine-and-cheese festival in the Arts District downtown a week ago and purchased a box of Richart® chocolates from Paris. No allergies. No drugs or tobacco.

Meds: oral contraceptive, MVI

Which of the following is the most appropriate next step in patient care?

   A. 100% high-flow oxygen through mask and counsel to refrain from alcohol
   B. CT of the head with contrast
   C. Ultrasound of the carotid arteries
   D. Verapamil daily
   E. Sumatriptan, single dose, and reassess in two hours

386.

A 58-year-old female presents complaining of a hand tremor that has been present for 2 years. Her family is concerned that she has Parkinson's. She notices the tremor daily. It rarely interferes with her functioning, but she is embarrassed in social situations. She notices that wine subdues the tremor, so she "always drinks at weekly sorority functions."

Which of the following is the <u>most</u> appropriate intervention?

   A. Chlordiazepoxide-weaning regimen for "gin fits" with follow-up in 4 days
   B. Propranolol
   C. Carbidopa/levodopa
   D. MRI of the posterior fossa
   E. Vascular evaluation of the posterior circulation

387.

A 23-year-old female with a history of epilepsy presents to your office complaining of severe nausea x 2 weeks. She states the nausea is so severe, she is sometimes unable to take her prescribed antiepileptic drug, carbamazepine.

Review of systems is negative. Her last seizure was 2 years ago. She otherwise strictly adheres to her medications.

No smoking or drinking.
Meds: oral contraceptive, carbamazepine, MVI
Exam is unrevealing.

Which of the following is the <u>most</u> likely cause of the patient's current complaint?

   A. Vertigo
   B. Pregnancy
   C. Benign neutropenia from carbamazepine
   D. Gallstones
   E. Delayed gastric emptying

388.

A 54-year-old male complains of episodes of dizziness (they last 25 minutes and resolve). He has been permanently dizzy since the last episode yesterday.

Diplopia
PMH: cigarettes and HTN
Exam: regular heart rhythm and no carotid bruits

Which of the following is <u>most</u> likely to result in the correct diagnosis?

   A. Transesophageal echocardiogram
   B. 3 sets of blood cultures
   C. Empiric treatment with meclizine
   D. Ultrasound of the posterior circulation in the neck
   E. Holter monitor

389.

A 27-year-old female complains of progressive weakness in the lower extremities x 2 weeks.
History of self-limited gastroenteritis 1 month ago
Afebrile
Normal cranial nerves
Motor weakness in hip and knee flexors
Decreased deep tendon reflexes
Normal sensation

Which of the following laboratory results is the <u>most</u> consistent with the correct diagnosis?

    A. Finding acetylcholine receptor antibodies in the serum
    B. Positive CSF PCR for *Borrelia burgdorferi*
    C. Positive serum RPR
    D. Elevation of protein in the CSF
    E. Positive Western blot for *Borrelia burgdorferi*

390.

A 70-year-old female complains of pain in neck, shoulders, hips, and thighs x 2 months. She has <u>not</u> been sleeping well and has noticed a 10-lb weight loss in 3 months.

Exam: normal strength.

Labs:
    WBC 9,500, normal differential
    Hgb 10.5
    Platelets 450,000
    Na 145
    K 4.2
    HCO_3 24
    BUN 12
    Creat 0.6
    Glu 92
    CPK 70 (50–170)

Which of the following is the <u>most</u> appropriate next step in management?

    A. Acetylcholine receptor antibodies.
    B. Anti-Jo antibodies.
    C. Low-dose prednisone daily.
    D. Peroneal nerve biopsy.
    E. Start pregabalin.

391.

A 27-year-old woman is brought to the emergency department by EMS after being found down by a neighbor. The neighbor states the woman did complain of a headache with some nausea but otherwise seemed fine. The patient does not use drugs, but she does drink wine daily and smokes cigarettes.

She has no past medical history and takes no medications.

Exam: T 98° F, RR 8, BP 100/65, HR 100,
BMI 19, oxygen saturation 97%
No response to sternal rub
Pupils equal and reactive
"Doll's eyes" present
Normal tone; no spontaneous movements
Toes down-going
ABG: pH 7.30, pO$_2$ 74, pCO$_2$ 60
Na 137, K 3.5, Cl 104, HCO$_3$ 27, BUN 25,
Creat 0.7, Glu 86

Which of the following is the most appropriate next step in patient care?

    A. Parenteral hydrocortisone tid
    B. Nasogastric tube and n-acetylcysteine
    C. Ceftriaxone 2 grams intravenously
    D. Naloxone
    E. Carboxyhemoglobin level

392.

An 18-year-old woman complains of a left, unilateral, throbbing headache that was preceded by "flashing lights in the right eye." The headache began at a wine-and-cheese festival, worsened over 30 minutes, and then persisted for 3 hours. The patient now complains of right hand and foot weakness.

Exam shows a mild right hemiparesis and word-finding difficulty.

PMH is negative.
Medications include an oral contraceptive pill and a daily multivitamin. No allergies. No drugs or tobacco.

Which of the following is the most appropriate next step in patient care?

    A. 100% high-flow oxygen through mask and counsel to refrain from alcohol
    B. CT of the head with contrast
    C. Ultrasound of the carotid arteries
    D. Verapamil daily
    E. NSAID and close monitoring of response

393.

A 48-year-old female presents to your office complaining of pain in her back and buttocks x 3 months. The pain is a severe ache, noticeable <u>most</u> often when she stands for prolonged periods. Pain is relieved when she sits or performs her daily exercise on an inclined treadmill.

Exam is normal.

Which of the following is the <u>most</u> appropriate next step in management?

A. Epidural steroid injection and bed rest
B. MRI of the spine
C. Analgesics prn
D. Referral to a neurosurgeon for laminectomy
E. Lower-extremity vascular evaluation

394.

A 48-year-old woman complains of "vision problems" which have gradually worsened over the past 6 months. She has no other complaints—no headaches, no weakness, numbness, etc. On exam, you find that she has diminished peripheral vision on both sides. You decide to order formal visual field testing to confirm this.

What is your leading diagnosis?

A. Cavernous sinus thrombosis
B. Pituitary tumor
C. Multiple sclerosis
D. Anterior ischemic optic neuropathy

395.

A 55-year-old woman has horrible stabbing/shooting pains in the left cheek when she eats or brushes her teeth. There is no associated weakness, numbness, fever, chills, nausea, vomiting, or concurrent illness. The symptom has been present for about 2 weeks; it has not been getting worse.

What is the <u>most</u> likely diagnosis?

A. Multiple sclerosis
B. Middle cerebral artery stroke
C. Tumor of the posterior fossa
D. Trigeminal neuralgia

396.

A 50-year-old man comes to the office with "clumsiness." It has been getting worse gradually over the past few weeks. At first, it involved the right foot. Later, he noticed problems in both feet and was "tripping over" his own feet. In the past week, he has noticed a change in his voice: It now sounds more "nasal." He denies recent infections. He has had no fever, chills, nausea, or vomiting.

On examination, he has a "nasal" sounding voice, but his speech is fluent. Naming and repetition are excellent. He has weakness of the legs more so than the arms. He has fasciculations of several muscles and is hyperreflexic in all 4 extremities.

What is the most likely diagnosis?

A. Huntington disease
B. Amyotrophic lateral sclerosis (ALS or Lou Gehrig disease)
C. Brain tumor in the dominant hemisphere
D. Herpes encephalitis

397.

A 78-year-old with hypertension and diabetes is admitted to the emergency department due to sudden onset of double vision earlier the same day. He denies troubles with weakness, sensory loss, or troubles with attention, concentration, thinking, or memory. On exam, he is unable to adduct the right eye.

What is the correct diagnosis?

A. Cerebral aneurysm
B. Right 6th nerve palsy
C. Left 6th nerve palsy
D. Internuclear ophthalmoplegia

398.

A 78-year-old man is brought in to your office by his daughter for evaluation. She was recently told by the patient that he converses with his wife for the last year, despite the fact that his wife died 5 years ago. She notes that he seems have difficulty accomplishing tasks he could easily accomplish before. For example, he could not remember how to shave once last week and called his daughter for help. She notes that on occasion he seems unable to care for himself and requires assistance from his family to perform some activities of daily living, but seems to function well the following day. The patient remarks that he enjoys talking with his wife and children as often as he can.

Physical exam reveals a thin older man in no distress. He is alert and oriented to person and place but cannot state the correct date. Neurologic exam reveals normal strength and reflexes. Gait is somewhat slowed. Mental status examination reveals impairment in drawing a clock and overlapping pentagons.

Which of the following is the most likely diagnosis?

A. Alzheimer dementia
B. Major depressive disorder
C. Delirium
D. Normal pressure hydrocephalus
E. Lewy body dementia

399.

A 34-year-old male presents to the clinic with complaints of unremitting and excruciating pain. It has been present for 2 years following a minor fall with bruising of the right thigh. He has been through several physicians and 2 pain clinics and states that he has been diagnosed with both reflex sympathetic dystrophy (RSD) and complex regional pain syndrome (CRPS). He is requesting extended release morphine, hydrocodone, and fentanyl patches.

Which of the following findings is <u>most</u> consistent with the diagnosis of RSD?

A. Abnormal reflexes in the affected limb
B. Atrophy of dermal components in the affected area
C. Characteristic abnormal findings on EMG
D. Dermatomal distribution of the pain
E. Elevation in the sedimentation rate

400.

A 56-year-old male with complaints of low back pain is seen in your office. Symptoms started 3 months previously when he was lifting some boxes and felt a "pop." The pain is in the left lower lumbar area and extends into the upper left leg.

On examination, the patient is tilting to the left side while sitting. His sensory exam of the lower extremity is inconsistent. His reflexes are muted. There is pain on left-leg raising that originates in the lumbar area and radiates to the left upper thigh.

Which of the following evaluation techniques is <u>most</u> likely to demonstrate a functionally symptomatic disk herniation?

A. Axial loading
B. Electromyelography
C. CT of lumbar region
D. Lumbar MRI
E. Lumbar spine series

401.

A 64-year-old female with chronic Parkinson disease is brought to the emergency department by her family because of an acute deterioration in her condition. She is confused, agitated, and diaphoretic. Her vitals include a temperature of 101.8° F (38.8° C) and a blood pressure of 192/108 mmHg. Remarkable physical findings include dilated pupils, hyperactive bowel sounds, and myoclonus with exaggerated reflexes.

Review of her medications includes a combination carbidopa/levodopa preparation, selegiline, amantadine, and fluoxetine, which were recently prescribed by her primary care provider. She has had no recent surgeries and has been fundamentally homebound.

Which of the following is the <u>most</u> likely cause of this presentation?

A. Neuroleptic malignant syndrome
B. Malignant hyperthermia
C. Anti-cholinergic toxicity
D. Serotonin syndrome

402.

You are asked to evaluate a patient who was admitted with complaints consistent with acute transverse myelitis. The patient has developed symptoms over the preceding 48 hours. Past history is remarkable for a one-day history 3 years ago of an acute vision disturbance. A diagnosis of optic neuritis was made at that time. Workup during that episode failed to establish an additional diagnosis.

Which of the following factors would be associated with the <u>most</u> severe prognosis?

A. Female gender
B. Relapsing-remitting cycles
C. Age of onset older than 50 years
D. Optic neuritis as initial symptom

403.

A 45-year-old woman presents with fever, irritability, headache, and meningismus. As part of the evaluation, a lumbar puncture is to be performed.

Which of the following is true regarding a lumbar puncture if the needle's stylet is removed during insertion?

A. The risk of developing an epidermal tumor is increased.
B. The ease of locating the spinal space is increased.
C. The risk of obtaining a "bloody tap" is decreased.
D. To avoid infection, once removed, the stylet should not be replaced.

404.

A 45-year-old woman comes to her clinic appointment with increasing symptoms of confusion over the past day, sweating, and increasing anxiety. She fell roller-skating yesterday and severely injured her shoulder (her R arm is in a sling). She has a history of depression, GERD, hypertension, and headaches.

Meds: omeprazole, lisinopril, metoprolol, citalopram, tramadol, and sumatriptan prn.
PE: Vs: BP 160/100, P 100
Tremor present, muscle rigidity

What is the <u>most</u> appropriate treatment?

    A. Dantrolene.
    B. IVF.
    C. Mannitol.
    D. Discontinue metoprolol.
    E. Discontinue citalopram and tramadol.

RHEUMATOLOGY

405.

A 75-year-old female presents with severe right shoulder pain preventing movement. She has a slightly bloody shoulder effusion with no crystals on polarizing microscopy. A radiograph shows calcific tendonitis and humeral head erosion.

The likely diagnosis is which of the following?

A. Crystal negative pseudogout
B. Rheumatoid arthritis
C. Milwaukee shoulder
D. Crystal negative gout
E. Humerus fracture

406.

Your patient, a 52-year-old, 70-kg woman with a diabetic nephropathy and a stable creatinine of 2.5, falls and injures her knee. Her orthopedic surgeon orders an MRI of her knee with gadolinium to assess whether she has torn her anterior cruciate ligament or her medial meniscus.

What is your appropriate response?

A. Perform a preoperative clearance assessment in anticipation of surgery.
B. Perform the MRI without gadolinium.
C. Add knee radiographs to the existing MRI order.
D. Replace the MRI with a bone scan.
E. Replace the MRI with a CT scan.

407.

A 57-year-old grandmother presents with 3 months of difficulty lifting her 2-year-old grandchild, difficulty initiating her swallow, and dyspnea with minimal exertion. Her laboratory evaluation revealed a CPK of 4,500. Her muscle biopsy reveals an inflammatory infiltrate comprised of lymphocytes and macrophages with muscle fiber necrosis and regeneration (consistent with polymyositis).

The additional evaluations of this patient should include which of the following?

A. Chest, abdomen, and pelvis CT scan
B. ANA, rheumatoid factor, ANCA, and angiotensin converting enzyme levels
C. Colonoscopy, Pap smear, mammogram, and chest radiograph
D. HIV, CMV, and herpes antibody levels; a hepatitis panel
E. Cervical, thoracic, and lumbosacral spine MRI

408.

A 62-year-old female patient with well-controlled rheumatoid arthritis takes methotrexate and adalimumab (Humira®). However, she wants to receive the shingles vaccine (Zostavax®).

How do you respond?

A. Yes, but because the patient is immunosuppressed, she will need a booster injection in a year.
B. No, because her medications prohibit her from receiving live-virus vaccines.
C. No, because patients with rheumatoid arthritis should never receive live-virus vaccines.
D. Yes, because all patients over the age of 60 should receive this vaccine.
E. It depends on whether this patient had chicken pox and her age when infected.

409.

A 62-year-old postmenopausal female with a history of hypothyroidism (for which she takes levothyroxine), severe GERD, and a recent radial head fracture is diagnosed with osteopenia (based on a T-score of −2.1).

In addition to prescribing calcium and vitamin D, which of the following treatment statements is true?

A. This patient does not require any additional therapy.
B. This patient is an ideal candidate for an oral bisphosphonate.
C. This patient is an ideal candidate for calcitonin.
D. This patient should receive yearly zoledronic acid.
E. This patient should decrease her levothyroxine dose.

410.

A 34-year-old male, with an 8-month history of arthralgias, is referred by his primary care physician because his laboratory studies were positive for RF and anti-CCP antibodies.

The anti-CCP antibody is associated with which of the following?

A. Early development of rheumatoid nodules
B. The development of a rheumatoid arthritis/lupus overlap syndrome
C. The development of a lupus nephritis
D. Early development of bone erosions
E. The development of amyloidosis of the kidneys

411.

A 28-year-old man complains of a 3-month history of morning lower back pain, lasting 2 hours. He also noticed a swollen left second toe for 2 months, has had pain in the bottom of both heels when he walks, and has a scaly skin rash along his scalp hairline.

What is the **most** appropriate initial therapy?

A. Etanercept
B. Methotrexate
C. Prednisone
D. Glucosamine
E. Celecoxib

412.

A 24-year-old female presents with 6 months of symmetric MCP, PIP, and wrist joint synovitis. Her ANA and RF are positive, and her hand radiographs do **not** indicate erosions.

Which of the following features suggests systemic lupus erythematosus rather than rheumatoid arthritis?

A. Her additional history of sicca symptoms
B. Her additional history of 3 miscarriages
C. Her additional laboratory finding of neutropenia
D. Her additional radiographic finding of bilateral pleural effusions
E. Her physical examination finding of synovitis

413.

A 26-year-old man presents with an acutely swollen knee. His aspirate contains cloudy fluid with 42,000 WBC (95% PMNs) and rhomboid-shaped weakly positively birefringent intracellular crystals.

The evaluation for an underlying cause of his condition should include which of the following?

CPPD

A. CBC, TSH, CRP
B. RF, ANA, dsDNA
C. Folate level, vitamin B_{12}, thiamine level
D. Ferritin, glycosylated hemoglobin, urate level
E. TSH, ferritin, calcium

414.

A 45-year-old male with a history of IV drug use presents with 3 months of lower extremity rash, fever to 101.0° F, 15-lb unintentional weight loss, fatigue, malaise, DOE, and progressive numbness in his feet. On physical examination, he has palpable purpura of his lower extremities. His laboratory studies include hemoglobin = 9.1, hematocrit = 27.2, and creatinine of 2.3 mg/dL.

What additional laboratory abnormality would you expect?

A. Elevated TSH
B. Positive hepatitis B surface antigen
C. Positive antihistone antibody
D. Lymphocytosis
E. Positive anti-myelin basic protein antibody

415.

A 55-year-old male presents with pain in the left groin with radiation to the inner thigh. He has no history of trauma. He drinks 2–3 six-packs per day of beer.

Musculoskeletal exam: normal ROM hips; pain in left groin with straight leg raises.

Hip radiographs: normal joint spaces, no osteophytes

Which of the following is the next <u>most</u> appropriate step in patient care?

    A. NSAID and rest followed by strength training.
    B. MRI L-spine.
    C. MRI bilateral hips.
    D. Inject the trochanteric bursa with a slow-release steroid such as methylprednisolone acetate.

416.

A 50-year-old female presents complaining of progressive weakness x 2 months.

She requires extra time to get ready for work because her arms tire while she is combing her hair, and she is unable to climb a single flight of stairs without stopping for rest. She denies fever and pain or swelling of any joints or muscles. She is otherwise healthy. Exam is normal at rest.

    WBC 9,500 (normal differential)
    Hgb 12.7
    Platelets 325,000
    Na 145
    K 4.2
    HCO_3 24
    BUN 12
    Creat 0.6
    Glu 92
    CPK 70 (50–170)

Which of the following is the <u>most</u> appropriate next step in management?

    A. Acetylcholine receptor antibodies
    B. Anti-Jo antibodies
    C. High-dose prednisone daily
    D. Peroneal nerve biopsy
    E. Colonoscopy

417.

A 70-year-old female with RA presents with new-onset lower back pain. She has received methotrexate and prednisone for the past 20 years. She requests permission to increase her current prednisone maintenance dose from 5 mg qd to her "flare dose" of 60 mg qd. Exam reveals RA deformities but without acute synovitis.

Her deep L-spine pain is <u>not</u> reproducible by palpation, and she has no pain with straight leg raises. No LE motor weakness or paresthesias. She denies groin pain.

Which of the following is the <u>most</u> appropriate next step in management?

    A. Increase prednisone to 40 mg daily.
    B. Start etanercept.
    C. Plain films of the spine.
    D. MRI of both hips.

418.

A 66-year-old female with HTN presents complaining of pain in her neck, shoulders, hips, and thighs x 2 months. She takes longer to dress in the mornings because of pain, and she is <u>not</u> sleeping well.

She denies weakness and swelling of any joints or muscle groups. Exam shows a 12-lb weight loss since her last visit 4 months ago, but she is otherwise normal.

WBC 9,500 (normal differential)
Hgb 10.5
Platelets 450,000
Na 145
K 4.2
HCO_3 24
BUN 12
Creat 0.6
Glu 92
CPK 70 (50–170)

Which of the following is the <u>most</u> appropriate next step in management?

    A. Acetylcholine receptor antibodies
    B. Anti-Jo antibodies
    C. Low-dose prednisone daily
    D. Peroneal nerve biopsy
    E. Pregabalin daily

419.

A 45-year-old male presents with a 3-month history of a tingly, lower-extremity rash, predominant lower-extremity joint pain, and a history of recent cold-induced color change of the hands.

CBC, LFTs, and U/A are normal.

Hepatitis panel:
  HAV +
  Anti-HBc IgM –
  Anti-HBc IgG –
  HBsAg –
  Anti-HBs +
  HCV +

Here is a picture of the rash:

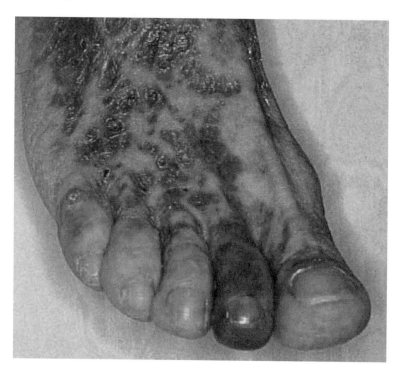

Which of the following is the <u>most</u> likely diagnosis?

  A. Meningococcemia
  B. Polyarteritis nodosa
  C. Immune thrombocytopenic purpura
  D. Wegener's
  E. Cryoglobulinemia

420.

Sausage digits with the additional finding of pitted nail beds are associated with which of the following inflammatory arthritides?

A. Rheumatoid arthritis
B. Sjögren's arthritis
C. Psoriatic arthritis
D. Reactive spondyloarthropathy
E. Ankylosing spondylitis

421.

A 45-year-old female presents with (R) long MCP swelling x 2 weeks.

Exam: inflamed (R) long MCP joint
Arthrocentesis: weakly positively birefringent crystals

Which of the following is the **most** appropriate next step in management?

A. Allopurinol.
B. Serum and urine uric acid levels.
C. Counsel to reduce alcohol intake and avoid foods high in purines.
D. Serum iron, TIBC, ferritin, TSH, and calcium.
E. ANA.

422.

Radiographs of a patient's hands show narrowed joint spaces of the DIP and PIP joints without erosions or chondrocalcinosis.

Which of the following is the **most** likely diagnosis?

A. Rheumatoid arthritis
B. Hemochromatosis
C. Osteoarthritis
D. Chronic polyarticular gout
E. Psoriatic arthritis

423.

A 45-year-old woman presents with intermittent wrist and hand pain for 3 weeks. She has a history of DM and HTN, and her medications currently include glyburide and a diuretic.

Exam: afebrile, R-wrist effusion without heat or erythema. She appears tan, and it is December in Minnesota.

Radiograph of her hand shows the following:

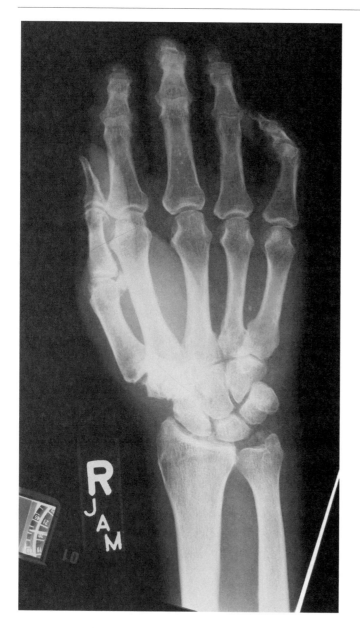

Which of the following is the <u>most</u> appropriate next step in patient care?

A. NSAID and wrist splint.
B. Serum uric acid level.
C. Iron, TIBC, ferritin.
D. Discontinue HCTZ and start enalapril.
E. ANA.

424.

You are called by nursing staff during the late evening for complaints of a patient who was admitted for neurologic symptoms following a fall from a tree resulting in head trauma and a fractured right forearm. He has been doing well for the previous 36 hours with improving mental status and was prepared to be discharged the following morning. His arm was casted earlier today after having been splinted for the initial two days.

The nurse informs you that the patient is complaining of significant pain in the right hand that has been increasing over the previous four hours.

Which of the following would be the _most_ appropriate next step?

    A. Request radiographs of the right hand.
    B. Ask orthopedics to evaluate before discharge.
    C. Titrate IV morphine to control the pain.
    D. Remove the right forearm cast immediately.
    E. Institute IV antibiotics after obtaining blood cultures.

425.

A 61-year-old woman with a hypothyroidism presents with 3 months of abdominal pain. The patient's pain is diffuse, worse after meals, is associated with nausea but no vomiting, and has been progressively worsening over the last 2 months. She was seen in an urgent care facility one month ago, diagnosed with _H. pylori_ by serology, and treated with triple therapy for _H. pylori_ gastritis. The patient has lost 20 pounds during this time. The pain did _not_ improve with treatment, and she comes in to clinic for follow-up.

A review of systems is significant for diffuse myalgias during this time. Fatigue and an episode of foot drop that occurred two months ago has since resolved. She has no diarrhea, melena, or hematochezia. Her past medical history is otherwise unremarkable; she is up-to-date with her routine health maintenance. She does _not_ smoke or drink alcohol and is _not_ sexually active.

Physical exam is significant for a blood pressure of 178/94, heart rate of 94, and normal oxygen saturation. The patient appears chronically ill; her heart and lung examination is normal. She has diffuse abdominal pain without rebound or masses. Her examination is otherwise normal.

Laboratory studies reveal a normal WBC, hemoglobin of 10.8, MCV of 82, normal platelets. Her ESR is 94. Urinalysis is significant for large blood, negative leukocyte esterase, and trace ketones. Urine microscopy shows 352 red blood cells/hpf, with 20 white cells/hpf.

What is the _most_ likely cause of the patient's symptoms?

    A. Resistant _Helicobacter pylori_ infection
    B. Nephrolithiasis
    C. Crohn disease
    D. Polyarteritis nodosa
    E. Colon cancer

426.

A 63-year-old female returns to your clinic for her annual physical examination. She is doing very well with her only ongoing complaint being chronic knee pain. Her condition has been diagnosed as osteoarthritis, and her complaints have been well controlled with acetaminophen.

Which of the following is the <u>most</u> likely side effect with this therapy?

    A. Gastroesophagitis
    B. Hepatitis
    C. Abnormal bleeding
    D. Constipation
    E. Glomerulonephritis

427.

Many arthritic processes are clinically very similar in presentation. Synovial biopsy can help provide diagnostic information in certain circumstances.

Synovial biopsy is <u>most</u> helpful in diagnosing which of the following arthritic processes?

    A. Tubercular arthritis
    B. Psoriatic arthritis
    C. Postinfectious arthritis
    D. Rheumatoid arthritis

428.

A 20-year-old male presents to clinic with knee pain. The patient is a college student and was playing basketball 3 days ago. He landed awkwardly, fell, and had immediate pain in his right knee. He was able to walk off the court on his own. The following day, he awoke to find his knee swollen and painful. He was able to walk, but was unable to practice and so is presenting to clinic.

His past medical history is remarkable for exercise-induced asthma.

He does <u>not</u> smoke, drinks on weekends, and is sexually active with one partner, with a lifetime history of 2 partners.

Physical exam is remarkable for a swollen right knee with a ballotable patella. The knee is <u>not</u> red or warm. He has no joint line tenderness. Lachman and anterior drawer testing are normal.

The next step in management of the patient is:

    A. Knee immobilization, rest, ice, elevation, and ibuprofen 800 mg three times a day
    B. Knee immobilization, MRI of the knee
    C. Knee immobilization, referral to orthopedic surgery
    D. Urine PCR for gonorrhea

429.

A 69-year-old woman presents with symptoms of severe muscle pain and joint pain. This has been present for the past 3 weeks. She has had no fevers, chills, or trauma. She has a past history of HTN, hypothyroidism, CAD, osteoporosis, GERD, and depression. Meds: omeprazole, metoprolol, alendronate, citalopram, levothyroxine.

What is the <u>most</u> likely cause of her pain?

    A. Citalopram
    B. Omeprazole
    C. Alendronate
    D. Metoprolol
    E. Hypothyroidism

430.

A 36-year-old man with a history of gout returns for follow-up. He has had a 2-day history of cough and fevers today. Chest x-ray shows a RLL infiltrate. PMH: CRI baseline Cr 2.0.

Meds: allopurinol 200 mg a day, colchicine 0.6 mg a day, citalopram 20 mg a day

Which drug would be <u>most</u> dangerous to prescribe?

    A. Azithromycin
    B. Clarithromycin
    C. Levofloxacin
    D. Erythromycin
    E. Chloramphenicol

431.

You see a 40-year-old woman for a first appointment. She has a 15-year history of arthritis and is currently on low-dose methylprednisolone. She has no other medical history and takes no other medications. She drinks no alcohol and never smoked cigarettes. Review of systems is negative for chemical exposures and recurrent infections.

Physical exam is remarkable for ulnar deviations of the fingers, warmth and swelling of the MCP and PIP joints, diminished range of motion of the small joints of the hands, and fullness on the left upper quadrant of the abdomen.

Laboratory results:
WBC:	2,100 cells/mm^3
WBC differential:	88% neutrophils
	10% lymphocytes
	2% lymphocytes
Hgb:	13.2 g/dL
Platelets:	277,000 cells/mm^3

Basic metabolic panel and urinalysis are normal.

Which of the following is the <u>most</u> likely diagnosis?

   A. Evan syndrome
   B. Corticosteroid-induced myelosuppression
   C. Felty syndrome
   D. Amyloidosis
   E. Gaucher disease

432.

You see a 70-year-old man for a routine exam. He is in excellent health and takes no medications. Family history is unremarkable. He drinks alcohol only occasionally and does <u>not</u> smoke. ROS is positive for nocturia (twice each night). Patient also has had occasional constipation and some hearing loss over the past year, but otherwise appears normal.

Physical exam:
   Healthy-appearing man
   Vital signs normal
   No lymphadenopathy
   Thyroid non-palpable
   Cardiac, pulmonary, abdominal exams normal
   No focal neurologic abnormalities
   No rash
   Prostate enlarged, symmetric, no nodules, nontender

Laboratory results:
AST:	30 U/L
ALT:	32 U/L
Alk Phos:	298 (36–92 U/L)
Calcium:	8.6 mEq/L
Phos:	2.2 mEq/L
Mg:	2.8 mEq/L
T. bili:	0.6 mg/dL
PT:	11.0 s
PTT:	20.8 s
T. protein:	6.4 g/dL
LDH:	80 (60–100 U/L)
Albumin:	3.9 g/dL
Urinalysis:	Negative
PSA:	4.2 (mildly elevated)

Which of the following findings is likely to be present with further testing?

   A. Extracapsular adenocarcinoma of the prostate on biopsy
   B. Cotton-wool appearance on skull films
   C. Elevated parathyroid hormone levels
   D. Elevated parathyroid hormone-related peptide levels
   E. Monoclonal spike on SPEP, increased uptake on bone scan

433.

A 35-year-old African-American woman diagnosed with diffuse scleroderma 2 years previously and followed by an outside provider presents to your emergency department complaining of severe headaches and flushing for 3 days. She was in her usual state of decent health until 3 days ago, when she awoke with a "pulsing" headache that has <u>not</u> resolved. The pain has reduced in intensity but episodically returns to a very intense pain. This morning she developed a nosebleed, which has never happened before. Review of systems is negative for nausea, vomiting, diarrhea, fevers, chills, and weight loss. She reports normal urinary frequency without flank pain or dysuria.

PE: BP 210/185, HR 98 bpm, RR 14, Afebrile
PE significant for obvious thickening of the skin on the face and sclerodactyly
Funduscopic exam shows normal retinas and no papilledema.
Non-displaced PMI, normal cardiac exam
Normal lung exam
No ulcerations on the fingers
No peripheral edema

Laboratory results:

CBC:	Normal
Na:	135 mEq/L
K:	3.2 mEq/L
Cl:	103 mEq/L
HCO_3:	23 mEq/L
BUN:	32 mg/dL
Creatine:	4.3 mg/dL
Creatine 3 months ago:	1.2 mg/dL
Albumin:	3.7 g/dL
LFTs:	Normal
Troponins:	< 0.01 ng/mL at 2 measurements 2 hours apart
Urinalysis:	SG 1.025, pH 6.0, protein 1+, blood none, glucose none, WBC 3–5, RBC 0

Electrocardiogram: Sinus rhythm with ST depressions 1.2 mm in leads 1, aVL, and V5–V6 consistent with LV strain. No hypertrophy is indicated.

Which of the following is the <u>most</u> appropriate pharmacologic management?

   A. Atenolol 50 mg PO now
   B. HCTZ 25 mg PO now
   C. Captopril 12.5 mg PO now
   D. Extended-release nifedipine 90 mg PO now
   E. Hydralazine 50 mg PO and isosorbide dinitrate 10 mg PO now

434.

A 25-year-old woman presents to your office for evaluation of a rash and muscle weakness for the past 6 weeks. On examination, you find proximal muscle weakness of the neck flexors, arms, and legs. She has a slight rash around her eyes and a scaly pink rash over her knuckles.

A biopsy of proximal muscle is likely to show which of the following?

A. Denervation changes
B. Immune complexes around muscle fibrils
C. Disappearance of muscle fibers
D. Malignant transformation
E. Fatty infiltration of muscle fibers

435.

A 24-year-old female presents with back pain. Although there is no specific history of trauma, she is on the gymnastics team and practices two hours a day. On exam, she indicates the pain is in the lower lumbar area. There is also evidence of tight hamstring muscles.

For which of the following conditions is this patient <u>most</u> at risk:

A. Slippage of the L5 vertebra relative to the body of the S1 vertebra
B. Loss of intervertebral disk height with associated disk herniation
C. Development of a spinal epidural abscess
D. Progressive development of lumbar scoliosis
E. Acute urinary retention or incontinence resulting from compromise of the sacral nerve roots

436.

A woman with long-standing scleroderma has significant finger deformities (pictured below).

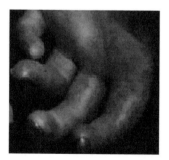

Which of the following explains this manifestation of her disease?

A. Cutaneous vasculitis
B. Digital tuft resorption
C. Inflammatory polyarthritis
D. Interosseous muscle weakness
E. Peripheral neuropathy

437.

A 68-year-old woman with a 30-year history of rheumatoid arthritis has been well controlled over the past 5 years using etanercept, methotrexate, and ibuprofen. She also has hypertension, "bone spurs" in her neck, diabetes, and is 15 pounds overweight. She noticed increasing pain and a creaking sensation in her left knee over the past 9 months. A standing radiograph reveals:

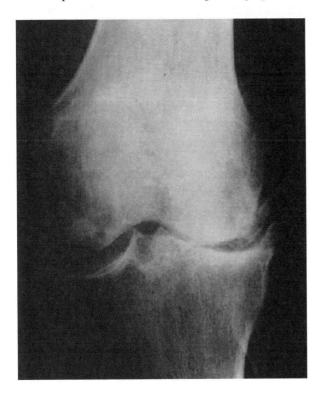

Which of the following is the <u>most</u> likely diagnosis?

    A. Complications of diabetes
    B. Obesity
    C. Osteoarthritis
    D. Osteoporosis
    E. Rheumatoid arthritis

438.

Hand involvement with osteoarthritis is common.

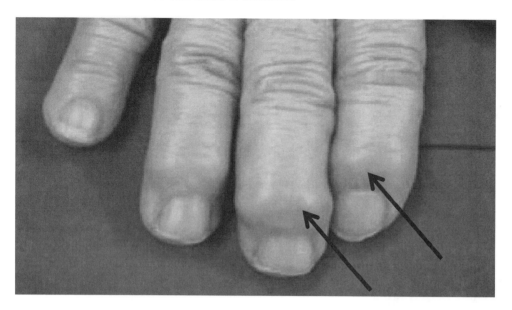

In this picture, what is the name given to the physical features identified by the arrows?

    A. Bouchard node
    B. Ganglion cyst
    C. Heberden node
    D. Rheumatoid nodule
    E. Tophi

439.

A 70-year-old female patient falls down the stairs and begins to have knee pain and swelling. She comes in for a knee x-ray one day later. She has never had knee pain or swelling in the past.

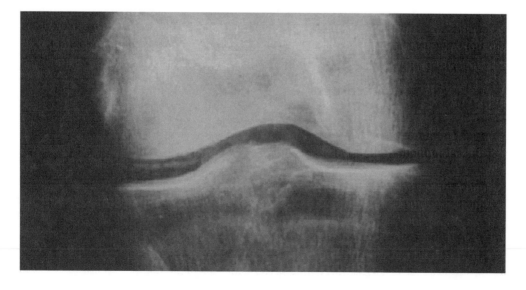

Which of the following can be diagnosed based on the radiograph?

A. Severe degenerative arthritis of her knee
B. Acute fracture of the distal femur
C. Healing fracture of the tibial plateau
D. Gout (uric acid deposition)
E. Pseudogout (calcium pyrophosphate deposition)

440.

Serologies are important aides in the diagnosis of diffuse inflammatory connective tissue disease.

Which of the following antibodies is matched with the correct connective tissue disease?

A. Anti-sclerotic 70 is associated with limited systemic sclerosis (also referred to as CREST).
B. Antihistone antibodies are routinely associated with renal disease in the setting of systemic lupus erythematosus.
C. RNP antibodies are associated with an increased risk of complete heart block in children born to patients with a history of lupus.
D. Anti-Sm antibodies are seen in approximately 25% of patients with SLE.

441.

A 54-year-old Caucasian male presents for evaluation of an acute painful right ankle. Symptoms began 24 hours prior to his visit. He has never experienced joint pain in the past. Other than being overweight and hypertensive, he is healthy. After unsuccessful trials of exercise and salt restriction, he was started on hydrochlorothiazide 6 months ago. There is no family history of arthritis. He recalls no injury.

Examination reveals: Temp 99.9° F (37.7° C), BP 160/92 mmHg, Pulse: 88 and regular, and RR: 12 and unlabored. Skin exam reveals no rashes or lesions. Cardiovascular exam reveals a regular rate and rhythm. An S_4 murmur is present. Pulmonary and abdominal exams are normal. Joint exam is significant for erythema and warmth of the right ankle. A small effusion is present. There is significant pain on attempted range of motion.

Joint aspiration reveals translucent fluid with the following characteristics:

WBC 4,500 cells/mm^3
60% PMNs
T. protein 4.0 g/dL
LDH 125 U/L (Serum 80 U/L)
Glucose 40 g/dL (Serum 95 g/dL)

Gram stain: no organisms
Polarizing microscope: negatively birefringent, needle-shaped crystals

Which of the following is the <u>most</u> appropriate management?

A. Draw a serum uric acid level to confirm the diagnosis.
B. Prescribe NSAIDs and allopurinol.
C. After treating his acute attack, consider switching his antihypertensive treatment from HCTZ to a different antihypertensive.
D. Exclude underlying etiologies by evaluating the following labs: TSH, ferritin, and calcium level.

442.

A 46-year-old male presents with a 3-month history of fatigue, low-grade fever, weight loss, and intermittent diffuse abdominal pain. Exam reveals a weak left foot to resisted dorsiflexion with altered sensation to light touch and mild abdominal tenderness with no rebound or guarding. There is significant tenderness on palpation of his left testicle.

Laboratory results:

HG:	10.9 g/dL
WBC:	10.8 cells/mm^3
PT:	508,000 cells/mm^3
BUN:	11 mg/dL
Creatinine:	0.8 mg/dL
Potassium:	4.0 mEq/L
Sodium:	141 mEq/L
Chloride:	102 mEq/L
CO_2:	24 mEq/L
LFTs:	Normal
Urinalysis:	2+Protein, 10–12 WBCs, > 100 RBCs, and WBC/RBC casts.
ESR:	120
RF:	positive
Cryoglobulins:	positive
ANA:	negative

Chest radiograph is normal.

Which of the following is the <u>most</u> appropriate next step?

A. Testicular biopsy for confirmation of diagnosis.
B. Initial treatment with 1 mg/kg/day of prednisone and plasmapheresis.
C. Screening for hepatitis A.
D. Begin plasmapheresis alone.

443.

A single 32-year-old male presents complaining of pain in both of his feet when he walks and discomfort with urination. He has no medical history and takes no medications. He is recently divorced and began a new sexual relationship with a woman 6 weeks ago. He does <u>not</u> use drugs or alcohol.

He states he was in his usual state of health until 5 days ago, when he noticed burning pain with urination but no trouble starting or stopping his stream. He denies any obvious urethral discharge. He reports that he and his new girlfriend do <u>not</u> use condoms during intercourse. Two days ago, he noticed pain in his heels while walking around the office. The pain has worsened such that now he can barely walk due to pain at the back of his ankles.

Given his current complaints, about which of the following systems should you inquire in conducting a review of systems?

    A. Joints
    B. Eyes
    C. Skin
    D. GI tract
    E. CNS

ALLERGY / IMMUNOLOGY

444.

You received an emergent call on the weekend from the wife of a 32-year-old male who was just stung by several wasps and is experiencing distress. She reports he has facial swelling, diaphoresis, lightheadedness, and difficulty breathing. A neighbor who witnessed the event had an EpiPen® and administered it to the patient. He was subsequently transported by ambulance to the emergency department. He received a dose of IV methylprednisolone and IV Benadryl®, and after 10 hours, his symptoms have significantly improved; the patient is being prepared for discharge home.

In addition to a prescription for an EpiPen, what is the next best step in the management of this patient?

- A. Prednisone taper.
- B. Diphenhydramine for an additional 24–48 hours.
- C. Referral to an allergist for immunotherapy.
- D. Albuterol MDI.
- E. No further action is necessary.

445.

Due to increasing symptoms occurring in individuals with latex allergies, latex-free gloves and bans on latex balloons are present in most hospitals.

Which of the following conditions has been <u>most</u> strongly associated with latex allergy?

- A. Nasal polyps
- B. Eosinophilic gastroenteritis
- C. G6PD deficiency
- D. Lumber yard exposure
- E. Spina bifida

446.

You are asked to evaluate a 27-year-old male who has been experiencing rhinorrhea and nasal congestion daily for the preceding 2 months. He is employed as a landscape assistant and works primarily outdoors. He has been using over-the-counter nasal decongestants that work well for him, but he is requiring increasing usage to control symptoms.

On examination, the patient has markedly edematous nasal mucosa. There is no purulence to the discharge, which is primarily clear in nature. There is no facial tenderness. Nasal smear is negative for leukocytes and eosinophils.

Of the following, the <u>most</u> likely diagnosis in this patient is:

   A. Allergic rhinitis
   B. Chronic sinusitis
   C. Rhinitis medicamentosa
   D. Vasomotor rhinitis

447.

A 23-year-old female comes to the clinic with complaints of vaginal irritation and swelling. She has had several episodes, which seem to be becoming more pronounced over time. She has been sexually active on four occasions with only one partner and states that she has used a condom and spermicidal each time. Symptoms began within hours of intercourse and persisted for four or five days. There was minimal discharge but some labial irritation and discomfort. She was unable to use tampons during this time due to significant vaginal discomfort.

On routine examination, there is normal female genitalia without redness or discharge. Bimanual palpation is within normal limits, and DNA probes and wet mount are obtained.

Symptomatic interventions and safe sex practices are reviewed with the patient.

That evening, the patient calls reporting that the symptoms have recurred. She denies intervening sexual activity. Contact with the lab indicates that results from the vaginal specimens are negative for evidence of STD.

The <u>most</u> likely diagnosis in this scenario is:

   A. *Chlamydia* infection
   B. Conversion reaction
   C. Latex allergy
   D. Sensitivity to spermicidals
   E. Toxic shock syndrome

448.

Your patient is a 26-year-old female who works as a carpenter. Over the last several years, she has experienced increasing breathing difficulties. Initially, she had a sensation of chest tightness on Mondays that would improve through the week, which she attributed to fatigue from the weekend's activities. The tightness, however, became more persistent and now lasts through the entire workweek. She has developed a recurring dry cough and has had several courses of antibiotics, but the cough has not improved.

The patient has good air entry in all lung fields but demonstrates both mild wheezing and significant expiratory prolongation. Chest x-ray reveals hyperexpansion but no masses or infiltrates. PPD testing is negative. PFTs show findings consistent with asthma.

Which of the following would help determine if this is occupational asthma or not?

   A. Perform a spirometry to determine this patient's response to bronchodilators.
   B. Give allergy shots, and if she improves, it was due to the wood dusts.
   C. Perform sputum washings to detect possible eosinophils or neutrophils.
   D. Perform skin testing to common allergens.

449.

A 25-year-old male presents with complaints of persistent rhinorrhea. The complaints started about 3 weeks ago, shortly after he began working at a local restaurant. His work requires alternating periods in the walk-in refrigerated area and the food-preparation area. The rhinorrhea has been clear and tends to be much worse at work. He has been taking various over-the-counter medications for allergies without dramatic response.

He has no facial tenderness. The nasal mucosa is boggy with increased erythema. No purulence is noted. The oropharynx is unremarkable, and there is no lymphadenopathy. Nasal secretions are clear with no purulence. No eosinophils or neutrophils are noted on smear of nasal secretions.

Which of the following would be the <u>most</u> appropriate therapy for this patient?

  A. Nasal steroids
  B. Oral decongestants
  C. An antibiotic course
  D. Oral antihistamines
  E. Nasal alpha-agonists

450.

A 23-year-old female returns to your clinic for a follow-up visit. She was previously seen when she developed bilateral difficulties with her pierced ears. She recently changed her ear studs and shortly afterward developed swelling and erythema to both pinnae. The ears improved with removal of all ear jewelry and 10 days of antibiotic therapy.

On today's visit, the ears are much improved. However, the patient has developed an irritating rash involving the left wrist and the lower abdomen. The wrist rash has a linear character and is so uncomfortable that the patient had to stop wearing her wristwatch. The abdominal rash is in the midline with distinct borders and is a circle approximately 1.8 cm in diameter. No other skin lesions are noted. Physical examination is otherwise normal.

Which of the following is the <u>most</u> likely diagnosis?

  A. Nickel sensitivity
  B. Köbner phenomenon
  C. Drug reaction
  D. Eczema
  E. Psoriasis

451.

A 26-year-old patient, who recently moved to the area, has complaints of eczema that has been recurrent since childhood but has worsened since the move to your community. The patient has used multiple interventions in the past with variable success.

Which of the following is the <u>most</u> appropriate pharmacotherapy?

    A. Prescribe tacrolimus cream (Protopic®) to be applied on the eczema.
    B. Prescribe low-dose oral steroids to suppress long-term eczematous symptoms.
    C. Advise patient to use soapy water to reduce skin irritants that cause eczema.
    D. Prescribe H_2 blockers to reduce the pruritus associated with eczema.
    E. Prescribe high-dose steroid cream to be applied where needed.

452.

A 44-year-old male presents with multiple vesicular lesions over both arms. He had been doing yard work in an overgrown wood lot. The lesions developed about an hour after he returned home and have been weeping since their appearance. The patient has multiple vesicular lesions, primarily in linear groupings. There is also some clean yellow "weepage" from some of the larger lesions. You suspect he might have been exposed to poison ivy.

Which of the following is the best next strategy for controlling the vesicular lesions?

    A. Advise the patient to avoid people because the serous discharge can transmit this disease from person-to-person.
    B. Prescribe a leukotriene inhibitor to prevent further vesicle formation.
    C. Carefully wash all clothing and tools from the work area to stop reinitiation of this rash.
    D. Prescribe steroids to keep weepage from becoming crusty.

453.

Identification of specific irritants can be very helpful in constructing an interventional plan for patients with severe allergies. Several testing modalities are available to help identify potential causes of allergic response. These include skin testing with standardized reagents and radioallergosorbent (RAST) testing.

Which of the following reflects the advantage of skin testing over RAST testing?

    A. Skin testing evaluates a broader range of allergic response mechanisms.
    B. Antihistamines do not interfere with skin testing procedures.
    C. Skin testing does not require trained personnel.
    D. Skin testing has a lower incidence of adverse reactions than RAST.

454.

You receive an emergent call on the weekend from the wife of a 32-year-old male who was just stung by several wasps and is experiencing a significant reaction. He developed facial swelling, diaphoresis, severe lightheadedness, and significant breathing difficulty. A neighbor who witnessed the event had an EpiPen® and administered its contents to the patient. His shortness of breath improved dramatically; his swelling reduced marginally, and his lightheadedness improved. His wife is asking for recommendations at this time.

Which of the following would be the <u>most</u> appropriate next step in patient care?

A. An oral dose of diphenhydramine, available in the patient's home.
B. Begin arrangements to have the patient seen by an allergist for desensitization therapy.
C. Call in a prescription for an oral steroid pulse, followed by a tapering regimen.
D. Call in a prescription for additional epinephrine with several refills.
E. Contact EMS for immediate transport to the nearest hospital.

455.

Your patient is a 36-year-old male who presents with complaints of "panic" attacks that have been increasing in frequency over the last year. He has experienced episodes of palpitations and flushing that come on unexpectedly and resolve after several hours. He has also had increasing crampy pain, primarily in the lower abdominal area, and frequent headaches. During this time, he has also developed recurrent swelling of his lower extremities with itching to the skin and the appearance of several reddish-brown maculae.

On physical exam, his vitals are normal. His cardiac exam reveals a regular rate and rhythm with no ectopy. His abdomen is soft with normal bowel sounds and no hepatosplenomegaly. He has several maculae on the lower legs with mild edema that seem to increase after initial palpation and become more pruritic.

Notable laboratory results:

Urine metanephrine:	83	24–96 mcg/24 hours
Urine vanillylmandelic acid (VMA):	6.7	2–7 mg/24 hours
5-hydroxyindoleacetic acid (5-HIAA):	20.1	0–31.4 µmol/24 hours
Tryptase:	82.4	2–23 ng/mL
C1 esterase inhibitor (C1-INH):	18.4	16–33 mg/dL

In light of the above information, which of the following is the <u>most</u> likely cause of this patient's symptoms?

A. Angioedema
B. Systemic mastocytosis
C. Carcinoid tumor
D. Pheochromocytoma

456.

You see a 28-year-old with a history of recurrent edema of the lips and face. She does not have urticaria with these episodes. She has come to the emergency department on numerous occasions, thinking she has had an allergic reaction; she is given epinephrine without any response. The edema gradually resolves over 1–2 days. Her brother and father have had similar episodes but are much less affected.

Which of the following is the <u>most</u> likely diagnosis?

A. Hereditary IgE hypergammaglobulinemia
B. Decrease in C1-inhibitor
C. Terminal complement deficiency
D. Atopic dermatitis
E. Arthus hypersensitivity reaction

457.

A patient with a known T-cell defect presents for routine evaluation.

Which clinical scenario is <u>most</u> suggestive of a T-cell defect?

A. Recurrent bacterial infections with encapsulated organisms
B. A history of frequent and recurrent episodes of otitis media, sinusitis, and pneumonia
C. Increased susceptibility to diarrhea as a result of infection with *Giardia lamblia*
D. Increased incidence of autoimmune disease—especially systemic lupus erythematosus
E. Recurrent and frequent infections with fungi, viruses, and protozoa

---

458.

A 27-year-old with trisomy 21 presents with weight loss, frequent diarrhea, and irritability. Abdominal distention and decreased subcutaneous fat are noted on physical exam. You suspect that he likely has celiac disease.

Because of its association with celiac disease, which of the following laboratory studies should you order?

A. Serum IgG antibody level
B. Serum IgA antibody level
C. Serum IgM antibody level
D. Serum IgD antibody level
E. Serum IgG subclass levels

459.

A healthy 26-year-old woman presents to your office complaining of "welts." She states that she exercises 4x/week, and, after she begins her exercise, her skin "breaks out in welts and itches." She is able to tolerate the rash and completes her exercise regimen, but she has intense skin itching for 30 minutes after exercise. Hot showers make the itching and welts worse. These irritating rashes after exercise have been occurring for 3 years now. She takes only multivitamins and has no medical history. She does not smoke or use drugs. She drinks alcohol occasionally. Review of systems is negative for nausea, vomiting, diarrhea, fevers, chills, night sweats, and weight loss.

Physical exam is normal.

Which of the following is the <u>most</u> appropriate next step in her care?

A. Measurement of complement levels
B. Measurement of erythrocyte sedimentation rate (ESR) and/or C-reactive protein (CRP)
C. Complete blood count with differential
D. Reassurance and suggest she take cool showers after exercise
E. Prescription of diphenhydramine before exercise

460.

A 26-year-old male with newly diagnosed Hodgkin lymphoma was admitted for workup and staging. On admit, he described severe dyspnea on exertion, and his hemoglobin was found to be 6.7 g/dL. He was typed and matched for two units of packed red cells and premedicated with acetaminophen 650 mg and diphenhydramine 50 mg. Thirty minutes into his transfusion, he develops fever to 102.5° F, shaking chills, and complains of subjective shortness of breath.

Physical exam reveals a febrile, slightly distressed male. BP 138/75, HR 110, RR 18
Pulse oximetry 98% on room air
Chest and lung exam are normal <u>except</u> for tachycardia and slight tachypnea
No skin rashes

The nurses call you to receive directions on whether to continue the transfusion. At the first sign of fever, per protocol, they stopped the transfusion and sent for the following labs:

WBC:	3,500 cells/mm³
Hgb:	6.4 g/dL
Platelets:	182,000 cells/mm³
Direct Antibody test (DAT):	Negative
Free plasma hemoglobin:	< 5 mg/dL (normal = < 5 mg/dL)

Which of the following is the <u>most</u> appropriate next step in patient care?

A. Ibuprofen 600 mg PO and meperidine 50 mg IV
B. Vancomycin 1 gm IV q 12 hours and ceftazidime 500 mg q 8 hours
C. Diphenhydramine 50 mg IV
D. Oxygen 2 liters via nasal cannula and furosemide 40 mg IV
E. Rapid infusion of ringers lactate and dopamine 2 mcg/kg/min

461.

A recently hired 66-year-old HIV-positive male nurse is referred to your office from the occupational health clinic at the local hospital for evaluation of his vaccination status.

You are able to obtain his vaccination records from the local county health department. He received all his childhood immunizations, including 2 doses of MMR when he became a nurse in the 1980s. His last tetanus booster, Tdap, was given 4 years previously. He self-reports having had clinical varicella at the age of 7 years. The occupational health clinic is concerned that he needs the varicella zoster vaccine because he is older than 65 and at higher risk for zoster.

Medical history includes diagnosis of HIV infection after a bout of *Pneumocystis* pneumonia 4 years ago, after which he has been adherent to his anti-HIV regimen. His last CD4 count was 190 cells/mm^3. Currently he is without complaints.

Which of the following is the <u>most</u> appropriate next step in patient care?

   A. The occupational health department is correct; he should receive zoster vaccine.
   B. Vaccinate him for MMR and pertussis using the new Tdap vaccine.
   C. Vaccinate him for MMR, Tdap, and varicella, because his original antibodies produced against varicella are likely impaired due to HIV.
   D. Do not vaccinate him for varicella zoster.
   E. Suggest that he quit working because he has advanced HIV infection, and he is likely to transmit opportunistic infections to patients. The need for vaccine is now irrelevant.

462.

A 27-year-old female G2P1 presents to your office as a referral from the obstetrician for evaluation of her RPR titer. Prenatal screening, performed at her first prenatal visit at 14 weeks EGA, revealed a positive RPR test with a titer of 1:64. Her confirmatory MHA-TP is positive. HIV ELISA is negative.

Medical history is significant for only penicillin anaphylaxis at the age of 7 after receiving a penicillin injection for pharyngitis. She describes a weeklong hospital stay and emergent intubation. She does not smoke, use drugs, or drink alcohol. She has no other medical problems and takes no medicines except prenatal vitamins. This is her second pregnancy.

She states she has never had syphilis before, and she is certain this is a new infection because she was tested for syphilis during her first pregnancy 2 years prior. Review of systems is negative for paresthesias, ocular changes, changes in personality/affect or speech, lower extremity weakness, or history of stroke.

Physical examination is normal except for a slightly enlarged uterus consistent with an early second trimester gestation. Pelvic examination reveals no evidence of chancre. Skin exam is normal.

Which of the following is the <u>most</u> appropriate next step in patient care?

   A. Hospitalize in the intensive care unit, then give benzathine penicillin G 2.4 million units IM once.
   B. Hospitalize in the intensive care unit, then give benzathine penicillin G 2.4 million units IM once per week x 3 weeks.
   C. Prescribe azithromycin 2 gm orally once.
   D. Order ceftriaxone 2 gm intravenously x 1.
   E. Arrange for penicillin desensitization and treatment with benzathine penicillin G 2.4 million units IM once per week x 3 weeks.

463.

A 37-year-old man presents with a history of recurrent sinopulmonary infections. He recovers from them fairly quickly, but he has between 5 and 7 episodes a year. Recently he received an infusion of packed red blood cells after a major motor vehicle accident. During the infusion he developed anaphylaxis. The blood bank and hospital checked for mismatch and found no evidence of incompatibility.

What is his likely underlying condition?

    A. Isolated IgA deficiency
    B. Terminal complement deficiency
    C. Systemic mastocytosis
    D. IgG deficiency
    E. IgD deficiency

DERMATOLOGY

464.

A 42-year-old housekeeper presents complaining of a 2-week history of an itchy rash under a ring she recently acquired. The ring is 24k gold, and she has not had any rashes on her wrists or neck where she also wears gold jewelry. There is no rash elsewhere.

What is the <u>most</u> likely cause of her rash?

A. Irritation from water trapped under the ring
B. Allergic reaction from cleansers she uses at work
C. Allergic reaction to gold
D. Localized atopic dermatitis
E. Allergic reaction to nickel

465.

You have been following a 28-year-old woman for several years for general health concerns and for persistent, cystic acne. She has not responded to topical retinoids or oral antibiotics. You decide to prescribe oral isotretinoin.

What is the <u>most</u> appropriate advice you can give her about childbearing?

A. It is safe to conceive while taking isotretinoin.
B. She should not conceive while taking isotretinoin, but it is safe to conceive as soon as the day after she takes her last dose.
C. She should be off isotretinoin for at least one month before considering pregnancy.
D. She should be off isotretinoin for at least one year before considering pregnancy.
E. She should plan for permanent sterilization after a course of isotretinoin.

466.

A 52-year-old man with past medical history significant for hypertension, diabetes, hyperlipidemia, and seizure disorder presents complaining of soreness in his mouth. On exam, you appreciate hyperplasia of his gingiva. His medications are phenytoin, hydrochlorothiazide, metformin, lovastatin, and fish oil.

Which of these is the <u>most</u> likely cause of his findings?

A. Hydrochlorothiazide
B. Phenytoin
C. Lovastatin
D. Fish oil
E. Metformin

467.

A 37-year-old man with a 10-year history of chronic plaque psoriasis was recently diagnosed with hypertension. You want to control his blood pressure without exacerbating his psoriasis.

Which class of medication may exacerbate his psoriasis?

A. Thiazide diuretics
B. Calcium channel blockers
C. Beta-blockers
D. Angiotensin receptor blockers

468.

A 46-year-old woman comes in for further workup after a skin biopsy by her dermatologist confirmed a diagnosis of cutaneous sarcoidosis. She is healthy in general and denies any shortness of breath. On examination, you note erythematous papules on her face and in a scar on her left arm. There are warm, tender nodules on bilateral shins.

Which of these findings portends a good prognosis for this patient?

A. Papules on the face
B. Papules affecting scars
C. Absence of respiratory symptoms
D. Absence of any ulcerative lesions
E. Nodules on the shins

469.

A 27-year-old woman with a history of severe acne presents complaining of drainage from the skin of her armpits and groin. On examination, you note fluctuant nodules on her scalp, atrophic ice-pick scars on her face, and communicating, draining sinuses in her axilla, inguinal creases, and perianal region.

Here is the axilla:

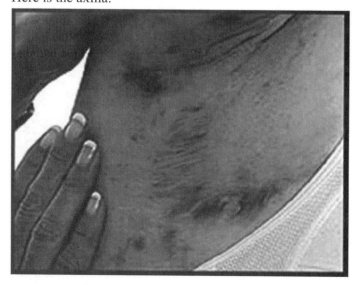

What is the <u>most</u> likely diagnosis?

    A. Hidradenitis suppurativa
    B. Furunculosis
    C. Pustular psoriasis
    D. Cystic acne
    E. Multiple epidermal inclusion cysts

470.

A 22-year-old woman comes in with follicular-based erythematous papules and pustules on her trunk. She reports the eruption is pruritic and began a few days after soaking in a friend's hot tub. On exam, the lesions are most concentrated in, but not limited to, the areas covered by her swimsuit.

What is the <u>most</u> likely causative agent?

    A. *Staphylococcus aureus*
    B. *Streptococcus pyogenes*
    C. *Neisseria gonorrhoeae*
    D. *Pseudomonas aeruginosa*
    E. Herpes simplex virus

471.

A 22-year-old man presents with a concern of a slightly itchy eruption on his chest, back, and arms. It has been present for months. He came in because it recently spread to his neck, and he is worried it will get on his face. He has not used any treatment. He has no family history of skin disease. Being an astute clinician, you perform a potassium hydroxide preparation from his skin scraping. Under the microscope, you see clusters of round circles and short, linear rectangles.

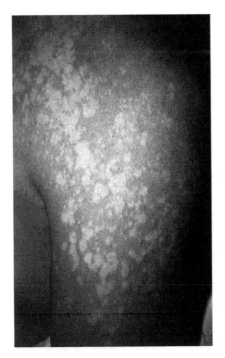

Scraping:

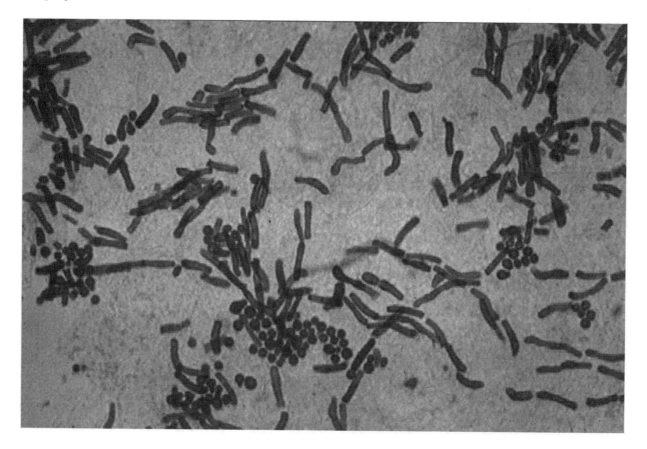

These findings <u>most</u> likely represent which of the following?

    A. Spores and hyphae of tinea corporis
    B. Spores and hyphae of tinea versicolor
    C. Eggs and droppings from scabies mite
    D. Eggs and droppings from body louse
    E. Diplococci of *Streptococcus*

472.

A 67-year-old man with past medical history significant for hypertension and hyperlipidemia reports 1-week history of tenderness on the right flank and 2-day history of blisters in the same region. Physical examination reveals a confluent, erythematous patch studded with vesicles on his right flank, extending from his spine to his umbilicus. The left side is unaffected.

Which of the following is the <u>most</u> appropriate treatment?

    A. Valacyclovir
    B. Bactrim
    C. Cephalexin
    D. Doxycycline
    E. Systemic corticosteroids

473.

A 44-year-old woman comes in for annual follow-up. While auscultating the patient's lungs, you note a 7 x 9-mm irregular, hyperpigmented papule with associated erythema. You are concerned about malignant melanoma.

Which feature of melanoma is the _most_ important in determining the patient's prognosis?

A. Asymmetry
B. Ulceration
C. Regression
D. Depth
E. Elevation

474.

A 26-year-old female presents with numerous rough, weeping erythematous patches in flexural areas of extremities and neck. This has been ongoing for several years, but worsened over the past week after she began using a new soap. She uses emollients and topical cortisone creams routinely.

What is the next best step in her treatment?

A. Oral antihistamines
B. Topical immunomodulators
C. Oral immunomodulators
D. Topical antibiotics
E. Oral antibiotics

475.

A 42-year-old obese male with a history of diabetes presents to you for evaluation of painful, moist, erythematous patches located within the abdominal skinfold. He noticed the skin rash during a visit to his sister in Florida.

Which organism is the likely cause?

A. *Staph aureus*
B. *Trichophyton* species
C. *Pityrosporum* species
D. *Candida*

476.

A 25-year-old man presents to your office for evaluation of a lesion on his leg. He states that he has had the lesion for more than 6 months. The lesion is rarely pruritic but is never scaly or suppurative, and now looks the same as when it originally formed about 6 months ago. He denies fevers, chills, weight loss, and bone pain. He has no other symptoms or similar lesions. He has not traveled outside of the United States. He religiously applies sunscreen during outside activities and denies ever having a severe, blistering sunburn.

Medical history is negative. He takes no medicines. He smokes a 1/2 pack per day of cigarettes. He drinks alcohol socially but denies drug use. Family history is noncontributory.

Physical exam reveals a 7-mm flesh-colored, papulonodular lesion with a shiny surface and a pea-like consistency on the anterior thigh without surrounding erythema. No other lesions are visible. Squeezing the lesion produces a dimple in the center.

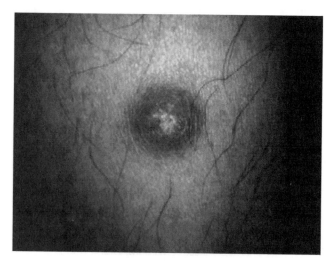

Which of the following is the <u>most</u> appropriate intervention?

    A. Observation only.
    B. Bone scan.
    C. Mammogram.
    D. Contrast tomography of the brain, chest, abdomen, and pelvis.
    E. Shave biopsy of the lesion for pathology.

477.

A 24-year-old male would like to initiate treatment for multiple, painful, tender, draining nodules, and inflammatory papules on the forehead, cheeks, chin, and trunk, which have been present for the past 4 years. He has been embarrassed by the appearance of his skin, but decided to see you due to formation of deep, atrophic scars.

The side effects of the oral medication used to treat this condition include which of the following?

    A. Epistaxis and xerosis.
    B. Arthralgias and headaches.
    C. Inflammatory bowel disease and hypertriglyceridemia.
    D. All of the choices are correct.

478.

A 30-year-old male presents to your office complaining of itchy persistent erythematous patches localized around the mouth and nasolabial areas. He denies any changes in his toothpaste, foods, or facial cleansers.

What is the best initial treatment for this condition?

A. Oral tetracyclines
B. Topical retinoids
C. Sunscreen
D. Emollients

479.

A 16-year-old male presents to your office with an acute diffuse, pruritic skin eruption with scaly 5-mm monomorphic plaques. Upon questioning, you find that the patient just returned from a Caribbean cruise, and that his girlfriend, who was also on the cruise, was ill.

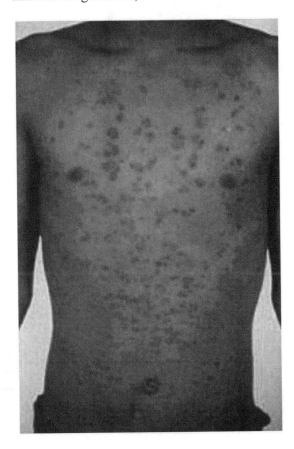

What is the likely cause of his skin eruption?

A. Sunscreen
B. Streptococcal pharyngitis
C. Arthropod bite
D. Either sunscreen or streptococcal pharyngitis

480.

You have been treating a 42-year-old African-American female for acne for the past 6 months with no improvement. She now has a cough and shortness of breath for which she would like antibiotics. Closer skin examination reveals violaceous papules located on bilateral cheeks and nose.

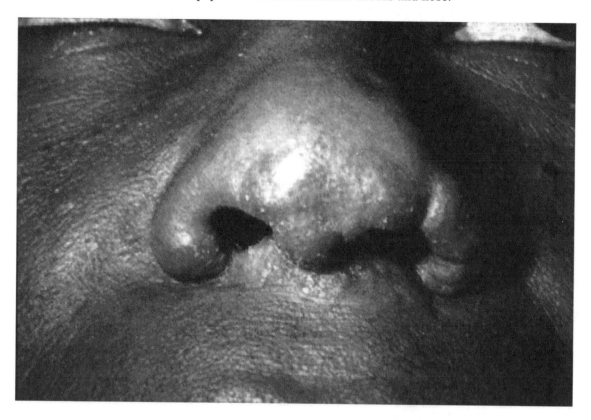

The next appropriate step in her management is which of the following?

    A. Prednisone for her skin and cough
    B. Chest x-ray
    C. Calcium and ACE levels
    D. Antibiotics to help her skin and cough

481.

You are seeing a 27-year-old female for well-demarcated, targetoid lesions on the upper extremities and hands. She states that the skin eruption started days after her cold sore appeared. She denies any fevers, cough, joint pain, or headache.

Which therapy is <u>most</u> appropriate?

    A. Acyclovir
    B. Doxycycline
    C. Erythromycin
    D. HPV vaccination

482.

A 63-year-old male kidney transplant patient of yours complains of a rapidly growing, tender, 2-cm nodule on the upper lip. He states that it started out as an ingrown hair that now interferes with shaving.

Which of the following statements are true of this tumor?

A. The metastatic potential is high.
B. The metastatic potential is low.
C. Family history plays a role.
D. Depth is the most important prognostic factor.

483.

One of your patients, a 30-year-old gay man, presents with purple papules and plaques on his trunk and buccal mucosa. These lesions are asymptomatic. You order a biopsy, which comes back positive for Kaposi sarcoma (KS).

Which of the following viruses is <u>most</u> likely related to Kaposi sarcoma?

A. Human herpesvirus type 1 (HHV-1)
B. Epstein-Barr virus (EBV)
C. Cytomegalovirus (CMV)
D. Human herpesvirus type 8 (HHV-8)

484.

You note multiple vesicles along a dermatomal distribution on the hemithorax of a 57-year-old woman. She has a history of varicella in childhood.

The following smear is performed:

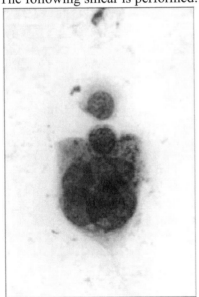

Which of the following would you tell this patient?

    A. The most likely etiology is herpes simplex type 2.
    B. The patient could present with this, even though she had not contracted varicella.
    C. The causative agent resides in the dorsal root ganglion of the spinal cord.
    D. One attack of zoster usually does not confer immunity.

485.

A previously healthy 28-year-old woman presents complaining of painful swelling in her hands and feet. She states that, typically, she does not have pain in her extremities, but she does notice swelling in both the hands and feet associated with decreased dexterity. When the weather is cold, however, her hands turn white, then blue, and are painful.

Review of systems is negative for skin rashes, joint pain or swelling, sexual activity, heart failure symptoms, and sleep apnea.

Past medical and family history is negative. She does not smoke or use drugs or alcohol.

Physical exam reveals a well-appearing female with obvious Raynaud phenomenon. There are no ulcerations. The distal skin on the hands and feet feel hard and thick with nonpitting edema. The upper arms and shoulders are normal.

She has many of the following lesions on her chest:

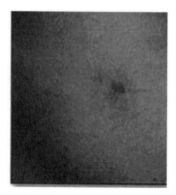

Other laboratory:
Anti-centromere positive
Anti-Scl-70 negative

For which of the following conditions is the patient at greatest risk?

    A. Pulmonary hypertension
    B. Esophageal dysmotility
    C. Interstitial fibrosis
    D. Malignant hypertension and renal failure
    E. Arrhythmia

OB / GYN

486.

A 35-year-old Hispanic woman presents for evaluation. She has done 2 home pregnancy tests, both positive. She has a rapid pregnancy test confirmed in the office today. On exam, her BMI is 30, BP 120/70, P 70. Fasting Labs: HbA1c 7.7, Glu 140, Na 140, HCO_3 28, Hct 36, TC 200, LDL 140.

What is her likely diagnosis?

A. Impaired glucose tolerance
B. Gestational diabetes
C. Type 2 diabetes
D. Type 1 diabetes

487.

A 24-year-old woman G1P0 presents 20-weeks gestation for follow-up. Her BP at work yesterday was 145/90. Today in the office, the BP is 146/93. She feels fine. A U/A is done and is normal.

What do you recommend?

A. Begin hydrochlorothiazide 12.5 mg daily.
B. Begin chlorthalidone 25 mg daily.
C. Begin losartan 100 mg daily.
D. Begin metoprolol 100 mg daily.
E. No treatment.

488.

A 25-year-old woman who received the HPV vaccine in the past has a routine Pap smear. All of her previous Pap smears have been negative. The results of this Pap smear show LGSIL (low-grade squamous intraepithelial lesion).

What do you recommend?

A. Repeat Pap in 6 months.
B. Repeat Pap in 1 year.
C. HPV testing.
D. Administer booster dose of HPV vaccine.
E. Refer for colposcopy.

489.

A young woman seeks your advice concerning her risk for having a child with achondroplasia. Her concerns arise because her brother has achondroplasia. Through a support group her brother attends, she met her fiancé, who is also diagnosed with achondroplasia. Both of her parents are of normal height.

Which of the following statements is <u>most</u> correct?

    A. Personally she has a 25% chance of being a carrier.
    B. Homozygotic children most commonly die in early childhood.
    C. All of her sons and half of her daughters should be affected.
    D. She has negligible risk of having an affected child.
    E. She has negligible risk of being a carrier.

490.

A 26-year-old renal transplant patient has been married for 2 years and is considering pregnancy. She had focal segmental glomerulosclerosis and received a cadaveric kidney transplant 5 years earlier. Her only problems since transplant have been hypertension and hypercholesterolemia. Her current medications are prednisone 5 mg/d, cyclosporine 125 mg bid, losartan 50 mg/d, and atorvastatin 20 mg/d. She became very anemic on both azathioprine and mycophenolate mofetil, so they were discontinued. Her BP is 118/64 mmHg, and her examination is unremarkable. Serum creatinine is 1.5 mg/dL; urinalysis has trace proteinuria.

Considering she may become pregnant, which of the following is the next <u>most</u> appropriate step in patient care?

    A. Stop her cyclosporine and increase her prednisone during pregnancy.
    B. Stop her losartan before pregnancy, and increase her prednisone when she becomes pregnant.
    C. Consider adoption instead of pregnancy because of the risk of rejection.
    D. Continue the same immunosuppressives, but stop the losartan and atorvastatin.
    E. Continue the same immunosuppressives, add hydrochlorothiazide, and stop the losartan and atorvastatin.

491.

A 29-year-old female patient that you have been treating for insulin-dependent diabetes mellitus informs you that she is anticipating having a child in the near future and asks for advice to improve the outcome of the pregnancy.

In addition to appropriate management of her diabetes and referral to an obstetrician familiar with high-risk pregnancy, what vitamin supplement is <u>most</u> important to recommend at this time?

    A. Vitamin C
    B. Folate
    C. Thiamine
    D. Vitamin D
    E. Vitamin K

492.

A 23-year-old female presents with complaint of irregular periods. She had menarche at the age of 12, and her periods were erratic initially. She later had several years of fairly regular menstrual cycles but then experienced progressively longer intervals between her periods. They are now very irregular, and the flow is unpredictable.

Initial laboratory results:

Follicle-stimulating hormone: 2.8 U/L
(FSH)

Follicular phase:	3.0–20.0 U/L
Ovulatory phase:	9.0–26.0 U/L
Luteal phase:	1.0–12.0 U/L
Postmenopausal:	18.0–153.0 U/L

Luteinizing hormone: 103.2 U/L
(LH)

Follicular phase:	2.0–15.0 U/L
Ovulatory phase:	22.0–105.0 U/L
Luteal phase:	0.6–19.0 U/L
Postmenopausal:	16.0–64.0 U/L

Estradiol: 1,598 pmol/L

Follicular phase:	184–532 pmol/L
Mid-cycle peak:	411–1,626 pmol/L
Luteal phase:	< 217 pmol/L
Postmenopausal:	< 184 pmol/L

Which of the following is the **most** likely diagnosis?

A. Premature ovarian failure
B. Polycystic ovarian syndrome
C. Prolactinoma
D. Asherman syndrome
E. Anorexia nervosa

493.

In November, a 34-year-old woman presents for primary care. She reports she is 25-weeks pregnant. She reports no history of chicken pox. She received all regular immunizations, with her last immunizations received prior to college 16 years ago.

Which of the following immunizations would be **most** appropriate?

A. No immunizations
B. Varicella, Tdap
C. Varicella, influenza
D. Varicella, Tdap, influenza
E. Tdap, influenza

494.

A G1P0 22-year-old woman presents acutely ill at 12 weeks with a 3-day history of vaginal bleeding, lightheadedness, fever, and chills.

On examination:

BP:	80/palpable
Pulse:	140/min
Temperature:	103.5° F (39.7° C)

Patient appears very sick, pale, and uncomfortable.

Laboratory results:

Hgb:	8.5 g/dL
Hct:	26.3%
WBC:	24,500 cells/mm^3 with 35% bands
BUN:	34 mg/dL
Creatinine:	2.1 mg/dL
Platelets:	190,000 cells/mm^3
U/A:	2–3 WBCs, many RBCs, 3–5 granular casts

She is immediately treated with IV fluids, packed RBCs, and broad-spectrum antibiotics. Twelve hours later, her BP is 104/76 mmHg, pulse: 116, and temperature: 100.4° F (38° C). She can sit up without feeling dizzy. Her serum creatinine is 2.9, and her urine output is only 10 mL/hour. She remains oliguric and requires acute hemodialysis for 7 days. After 7 days, her urine output increases, and her serum creatinine eventually falls to 1.1 mg/dL.

Which of the following is the <u>most</u> likely cause of her renal failure?

    A. Acute cortical necrosis
    B. Acute tubular necrosis
    C. Preeclampsia
    D. Prerenal azotemia
    E. Rhabdomyolysis

495.

You are asked to evaluate a 25-year-old patient on the obstetrics floor who is in the 33rd week of her second pregnancy. She has experienced significant elevations of blood pressure and increasing levels of protein in her urine.

Laboratory testing includes:

Hgb:	9.5	12.5–15.3 g/dL
Hct:	29.8	36–48%
WBC:	10.8	4.5–11.0 10^3/mm^3
Platelets:	88	150–350 10^3/mm^3
SGOT (AST):	138	0–40 U/L
SGPT (ALT):	143	2–45 U/L

Which of the following is the **most** appropriate next step in management?

A. Prompt delivery of her child
B. Transfusion of packed RBCs and platelets
C. Plasmapheresis
D. Intravenous glucocorticoids

496.

Your patient is a 65-year-old female with a history of repetitive episodes of dysuria and vaginal pruritus. During the last several months, she has sought care in several local urgent care clinics. With these visits, she has received several courses of antibiotics and has had multiple urine cultures, all of which failed to demonstrate a significant pathogen.

On her visit today, the patient also complains of increasing dyspareunia. Her last menstrual period was 13 years ago.

A pelvic examination is performed and reveals thin vaginal mucous membranes with some light bleeding associated with speculum contact. There is no significant discharge. Probes for gonorrhea and *Chlamydia* are taken; specimen for wet mount is collected, and urine is obtained for culture.

Results for *Chlamydia* and gonorrhea are negative. Wet mount demonstrates parabasal cells but otherwise is unremarkable. Urine culture shows mixed flora with no predominant organism.

Which of the following is the **most** appropriate intervention at this time?

A. Topical estrogen
B. Intramuscular ceftriaxone
C. Oral doxycycline
D. Oral metronidazole
E. Topical clotrimazole

497.

A 27-year-old female presents to the emergency department following the dysfunction of a condom during intercourse. She states that she uses oral contraceptive pills but frequently misses doses and thinks she may have skipped 3 pills in the last ten days. Her last menstrual period was 13 days ago but was shorter than normal. She is adamant that she does not want a pregnancy at this time.

Which of the following is a contraindication to using emergent hormone contraception?

A. Negative serum pregnancy test
B. Positive urine pregnancy test
C. Concurrent usage of an oral retinoid
D. Irregular compliance with a triphasic oral contraceptive

498.

You see a 66-year-old Caucasian female in your office for routine care. She is well and has not been in for a clinic visit in more than 2 years. She continues to smoke 5–10 cigarettes/day and is relatively active. Her sister recently experienced a hip fracture, and she is concerned about her personal risk for osteoporosis. As part of your evaluation, you discuss the option of a bone density scan.

Which of the following is consistent with bone density testing?

    A. A positive T-score indicates a bone density less than young healthy individuals.
    B. A negative Z-score indicates a bone density higher than sex-matched, age-controlled peers.
    C. A normal bone density noted on routine x-ray eliminates the need for bone density studies.
    D. Results of bone density scans performed by different techniques are difficult to directly compare.

499.

You evaluate a 26-year-old woman for pelvic inflammatory disease.

Which of the following signs or symptoms represent the <u>minimum</u> criteria needed to initiate empiric treatment for pelvic inflammatory disease in a sexually active patient?

    A. Uterine/adnexal tenderness or cervical motion tenderness
    B. Mucopurulent cervical discharge or presence of white blood cells on wet prep exam
    C. Increased C-reactive protein or increased erythrocyte sedimentation rate
    D. Elevated temperature or elevated white blood cell count
    E. Documented infection with *Neisseria gonorrhoeae* or *Chlamydia trachomatis* within the past 3 months

500.

Which of the following associated findings requires hospitalization of a patient with pelvic inflammatory disease (PID), as opposed to initiation of outpatient treatment?

    A. HIV positivity
    B. Tuboovarian abscess in the differential diagnosis
    C. Culture positivity for both *N. gonorrhoeae* and *Chlamydia*
    D. History of PID 2 years previously
    E. History of pregnancy 9 months ago

501.

A 25-year-old woman presents to the emergency department with complaints of increased temperature, nausea, vomiting, and moderate-to-severe right upper quadrant pain. She completed a normal menstrual period two days prior to presentation. She has been on oral contraceptives for the last 6 months. On physical exam, she is noted to have generalized abdominal pain, which is worse in the right upper quadrant along with vaginal discharge and cervical motion tenderness.

What is the <u>most</u> likely diagnosis?

    A. Peritonitis associated with a ruptured ovarian cyst
    B. Acute cholelithiasis
    C. Ectopic pregnancy
    D. Perihepatitis
    E. Perforated appendicitis

OPHTHALMOLOGY

502.

A 32-year-old man presents to your office complaining of a painful rash on his forehead and nose, which first began as pain and tingling and progressed to blister formation over 24 hours. He now has unrelenting pain on the left side of his face and some irritation in the left eye. He believes he got an eyelash hair in his eye, and he is unable to remove it. Past medical history is remarkable for HIV infection with a recent CD4 count of 100 cells/mm^3. He has never had these symptoms before. He has been hospitalized with *Pneumocystis* pneumonia (PCP) and disseminated histoplasmosis in the past. He denies recent drug use or new sexual contacts.

Medications include Combivir®, tenofovir, lopinavir-ritonavir, trimethoprim/sulfamethoxazole, and itraconazole. He says he is "somewhat adherent" to his medications, often missing evening doses.

Physical exam reveals painful, clear vesicles on the left side of the forehead and on the tip of the nose, with surrounding erythema. The left conjunctiva is slightly hyperemic but without obvious lesions or foreign bodies. Examination of the cornea with fluorescein dye reveals no obvious ulcerations. The remainder of the physical examination is normal.

Which of the following is the <u>most</u> appropriate pharmacotherapy?

    A. Hospital admission for intravenous amphotericin B deoxycholate
    B. Oral acyclovir + intraocular trifluridine drops
    C. Oral acyclovir + intraocular trifluridine drops + intraocular dexamethasone
    D. Hospital admission for intravenous acyclovir at a dose of 3 mg/kg
    E. Hospital admission for intravenous acyclovir at a dose of 10 mg/kg

503.

An otherwise healthy 50-year-old man presents to your office complaining of a headache and right eye pain for 2 days. He states that his 10-year-old daughter recently developed "a cold" with symptoms of runny nose and a slight cough. Her eye became red and "matted," and she was given topical antibiotics by her pediatrician. He began taking pseudoephedrine because of some early symptoms of nasal stuffiness, and yesterday he noticed a slight redness in his right eye. He began using his daughter's topical antibiotics without improvement. Over the past 24 hours, the pain in his eye is worsening, and he has developed an unrelenting "boring" headache. Review of systems is positive for occasional blurry vision and "a fuzziness around the lights," which he most commonly experiences at night, but he is not currently experiencing these symptoms.

He takes no medications and sees a physician yearly for a routine physical exam and general screening. He does not use tobacco, drugs, or alcohol.

On physical examination, there is right scleral injection. The ocular movements are intact. On acuity testing in the right eye, he is able to identify only gross hand movements, but not individual fingers, and he has no peripheral vision. You are unable to perform a funduscopic examination because of his discomfort. There is a right mid-dilated pupil.

Which of the following is the <u>most</u> likely diagnosis?

   A. Acute angle-closure glaucoma
   B. Subarachnoid hemorrhage
   C. Fusarium keratitis
   D. Cluster headache
   E. Adenoviral conjunctivitis

504.

An otherwise healthy 50-year-old man presents to your office complaining of a headache and right eye pain for 2 days. He began taking pseudoephedrine because of some early symptoms of nasal stuffiness, and yesterday he noticed a slight redness in his right eye. Over the past 24 hours, the pain in his eye is worsening, and he has developed an unrelenting "boring" headache. Review of systems is positive for occasional blurry vision and episodes of seeing "fuzzies" around lights. These symptoms usually occur at night, but he is not experiencing them currently.

He takes no medications and sees a physician yearly for a routine physical exam and general screening. He does not use tobacco, drugs, or alcohol.

On physical examination, there is right scleral injection. The ocular movements are intact. On acuity testing in the right eye, he is able to identify only gross hand movements, but not individual fingers, and he has no peripheral vision. You are unable to perform a funduscopic examination because of his discomfort. There is a right mid-dilated pupil.

Which of the following is the next step in patient care?

   A. Intraocular dexamethasone
   B. Oral prednisone
   C. Intraocular gentamicin
   D. Emergent referral to an ophthalmologist
   E. Contrasted tomography of the brain

505.

A 24-year-old female presents to your office complaining of left eye tearing and redness for 1 day. She states she was in her normal state of good health until 3 days ago, when she began having nasal congestion and a sore throat. The rhinorrhea has continued, but the sore throat has improved. On day 3, she noticed upon awakening that her left eye was slightly irritated, but there was no frank pain. Throughout the day, she noted increased tearing, but no change in discomfort. She denies any colored ocular discharge or trauma to the eye. Review of systems is negative. She denies tobacco, alcohol, or drugs. She wears contact lenses and swims daily at the local YMCA outdoor pool.

Limited physical exam: bilaterally equal and reactive pupils, injected conjunctiva in the left eye, no photophobia, normal extraocular movements, clear tearing, acuity testing 20/15 in both eyes with glasses, and clear rhinorrhea

Her eye is shown below:

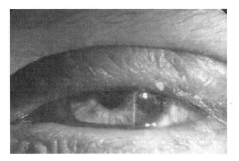

Which of the following is the <u>most</u> effective management?

A. Fluorescein stain to assess for an occult foreign body
B. Intraocular erythromycin
C. Intraocular ciprofloxacin
D. Reassurance with continued temporary abstinence from contact lens wear
E. Immediate referral to an ophthalmologist

506.

A 72-year-old female presents to your office for her yearly examination. Her past medical history includes stable hypertension, for which she takes atenolol and hydrochlorothiazide, and diet-controlled hyperlipidemia. She has no complaints. In review of systems, she admits to occasional episodes of burning pain on the left side of her forehead, which occurs twice weekly and are now increasing in frequency. She states she is unable to wear her hat while picking pecans in her yard, because the hat irritates her forehead. Sometimes, she notices the same burning radiating into her left jaw, especially when eating crunchy vegetables. She does feel more tired than usual, which she attributes to getting older. Last week, after working particularly hard in the yard on a hot day, she felt dizzy and noticed severe blurring of her vision, all of which improved with rest and has not reoccurred. On examination of her vital signs, you realize she has lost 30 pounds in the last year. She says she is eating less, because she does not have much of an appetite.

Her physical examination is normal.

Laboratory results:
    WBC: 8.5 cells/mm^3
    Hematocrit: 43%
    Platelets: 580,000 cells/mm^3
    Erythrocyte sedimentation rate: 110 mm

For which of the following conditions is this patient at greatest risk?

A. Bilateral blindness
B. Herpes zoster ophthalmicus
C. Metastasis of malignancy
D. Cerebrovascular accident
E. Presbycusis

507.

You receive a referral of a 30-year-old African-American female from the local emergency department, where she was seen 4 days ago and was told she probably has Lyme disease. She received a follow-up phone call today from the emergency department saying her Lyme test is positive. She was referred to both your office and an ophthalmologist, whom she saw this morning.

She reports being in a good state of health until 6 months ago, when she began feeling tired. She has gradually become more short of breath and developed a nonproductive cough for the past 3 months. In the last week, she has developed 2 disturbing symptoms for which she presented to the emergency department: Both of her ankles have become swollen and tender, and she has pain, redness, and excess tearing of her left eye.

She is married and does not use drugs or alcohol. She has no significant medical history and lives in Denver, where she works as a journalist for the *Denver Times*. She covers local stories and has not traveled much in her life. Specifically, she has not been to the northeastern U.S., the upper Midwest, or California. Review of systems is negative for hemoptysis, orthopnea, paroxysmal nocturnal dyspnea, wheezing, alopecia, miscarriages, facial rashes, recent change in sexual partners, history of syphilis or TB exposures, or weight loss.

The ophthalmologist diagnosed her with anterior uveitis, prescribed intraocular steroid drops, and encouraged her to keep her appointment with you.

Physical examination:
Normal vital signs
Eye exam: Unilateral conjunctival injection with direct and consensual photophobia
             Reduced acuity in the affected eye
             Normal ocular movements

No skin rashes are noted.
Normal jugular venous pressure and pulsations
Symmetric lung expansion with scattered, fine crackles throughout the fields
Both ankles are swollen and painful, without erythema. Other joints are normal.

Other results from the emergency department:
RPR nonreactive
HIV rapid screen negative
Lyme ELISA IgG positive
ANA negative

Which of the following is <u>most</u> likely to confirm the correct diagnosis?

    A. PPD placement
    B. Chest radiograph
    C. Colonoscopy
    D. *Borrelia burgdorferi* Western blot
    E. Sacroiliac joint films

508.

A 40-year-old HIV-positive man presents to your office complaining of seeing lightning spots. He has seen an infectious disease specialist for his HIV and states he is doing "well" with a recent CD4 count of 475 cells/mm^3 and good adherence to his HAART regimen. He has no history of AIDS-defining illnesses; however, he does have a long history of crack cocaine abuse from which he has been abstinent from until he began using again 3 weeks ago.

He reports being arrested 4 days ago for buying drugs on a street corner, and during the arrest, he ran from the police officer, tripped on a hole, and hit the left side of his forehead on a log. He denies having lost consciousness. He made bail, and shortly thereafter, began seeing flashes of light in his left eye. Last night, he noticed floating objects start at the rim of his vision at 9 o'clock and proceed in a circular pattern to 12 o'clock. He has always experienced floaters, but never in this specific pattern. He denies eye pain, excessive lacrimation, foreign body sensations, redness, or reduced visual acuity. He has been wearing glasses for nearsightedness since he was 15 years old. Review of systems is otherwise negative. He has not seen an ophthalmologist in the past 3 years.

Physical examination is normal.

He says he needs you to complete your recommendations quickly because he has "business to attend to," and he refuses to wait while you consult with his HIV physician.

Which of the following is the <u>most</u> appropriate next step in patient care?

    A. Initiation of valganciclovir 900 mg PO bid with food and urgent ophthalmologic referral
    B. Referral to an ophthalmologist for evaluation within the week
    C. Initiation of sumatriptan succinate as needed for symptoms
    D. Emergent lumbar puncture
    E. Referral to an ophthalmologist for evaluation today

509.

A 26-year-old man presents to the emergency department complaining of progressive vision loss in his right eye. He reports a decline in his general health over the past year with a 50-lb weight loss and subjective fevers at night 3x/week. Of late, he's noticed a variety of skin rashes that come and go on his trunk and upper extremities. The most recent rash is described as "itchy, red bumps."

He began to notice blurriness of his vision 3 months ago when attempting to redesign the website for his floral business. Over time, he has lost the ability to see intricate floral structures. This week, he believes he is losing his ability to distinguish colors, and he now has blurriness in his left eye. He has never had pain, redness or tearing, nor has he experienced any trauma. He specifically denies seeing flashes of light or large black holes in his visual fields. He admits to seeing occasional floaters of no specific pattern.

He has no significant past medical history but admits he does not go to the doctor "unless I'm about to die." He lives alone and is not married. He smokes 1/2 pack of cigarettes per day but denies use of alcohol or drugs. He owns two inside cats.

Physical exam reveals a cachectic male with normal vital signs. Eye exam is significant for a normal-appearing eye with reduced visual acuity (can distinguish waving objects only, not count fingers) and normal ocular motions. Funduscopic evaluation of both eyes shows fluffy white infiltrates and multiple retinal hemorrhages, although the right eye is worse. There is no excess tearing or photophobia. A pruritic, pinpoint, erythematous rash covers both arms. The remaining neurologic exam is normal.

Which of the following is the <u>most</u> appropriate next step in patient care?

    A. CMV IgM titer
    B. *Bartonella henselae* IgG and IgM titers
    C. HIV ELISA test
    D. Ganciclovir 5 mg/kg IV q 12 hours
    E. Penicillin 18–24 mU/day IV x 10–14 days

510.

A 40-year-old woman presents complaining of itchy eyes. She states that she has had problems with her eyes feeling "scratchy" for at least 2 years now, and she attributes this to having just moved to the southern climate and developing allergies. She has taken diphenhydramine without relief, and she asks for a prescription medication to help with allergy symptoms. She does notice that artificial tears help. Review of systems is positive only for occasional trouble swallowing, especially if eating breaded foods such as crackers. She has no medical history and takes no medications. Her mother and father are alive and well, and she has no siblings. She denies drugs and alcohol and tobacco use.

On examination, you notice bilateral parotid and submandibular gland swelling, and there is conjunctival injection. The remainder of the physical exam is normal.

Ophthalmology consultation reveals a normal slit lamp examination with a Schirmer tear test result = 2 mm (abnormal). Diagnosis: "keratoconjunctivitis sicca."

Laboratory results:
    CBC: normal
    Anti-SSA/Ro and Anti-SSB/La: positive
    Rheumatoid Factor: positive
    Lip gland biopsy shows focal collections of lymphocytes

For which of the following conditions is the patient at greatest risk?

    A. Erosive arthritis
    B. Non-Hodgkin lymphoma
    C. Pulmonary hypertension
    D. Cataracts
    E. Stroke

511.

A 42-year-old man presents to the emergency department complaining of reduced vision in his left eye, as well as fevers. He has no significant past medical history and does not see physicians routinely. He is a construction worker and admits to injecting methamphetamine intravenously at least 3x weekly. He states he does not share needles, but he does reuse the same needle repeatedly. Last week, one of the needles broke off into his forearm during an injection. He reports no pain or erythema at that site. However, 4 days later, he began experiencing bouts of fever with shaking chills. He has no appetite and feels generally ill. Review of systems is positive for nausea and anorexia. Over the past 24 hours, he has noticed a progressive decrease in vision in his left eye, with parts of the visual fields completely obscured.

He prepared his drug to be injected by dissolving the solid methamphetamine in lemon juice. He purchases the pre-squeezed juice, stored in the small lemon-shaped bottles, from the grocery store. He reports purchasing a new bottle last week.

Physical examination: Temperature: 101.5° F (38.6° C), HR: 110, BP: 117/65 mmHg, normal respirations

Generally, he appears ill. Limited bedside funduscopic examination reveals multiple, whitish chorioretinal spots.

Which of the following is the <u>most</u> appropriate next step in diagnosis?

A. Vitrectomy with culture of vitreous fluid
B. HIV ELISA test
C. Excision and culture of embedded needle
D. Aerobic, anaerobic, and fungal blood cultures
E. Lumbar puncture with testing for cryptococcal antigen

512.

A 59-year-old man presents to the emergency department with sudden vision loss. He denies any pain.

On ophthalmologic examination, you note the following:

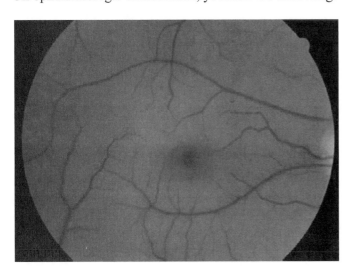

What is the <u>most</u> likely diagnosis?

    A. Retinal detachment
    B. Retinal artery occlusion
    C. Retinal vein occlusion
    D. Endophthalmitis
    E. Occipital cortex infarct

513.

A 66-year-old male presents to the clinic with a painful rash on his nose and irritation and discomfort in his left eye. He denies any trauma or exposures. The rash is located on the left side of the nose with some extension onto the cheek. The lesions are vesicular with surrounding erythema and light yellow crusting. There is diffuse redness to the conjunctiva, and a fluorescein examination demonstrates frond-like lesions.

After consultation with an ophthalmologist, which of the following is the <u>most</u> appropriate therapy for this patient's conjunctivitis?

    A. Ciprofloxacin
    B. Acyclovir
    C. Prednisone
    D. Erythromycin

PSYCHIATRY

514.

You are called to evaluate a 68-year-old man with a past history of hyperlipidemia and hypertension treated with hydrochlorothiazide. He was hospitalized for a left hip fracture that was repaired 3 days ago and was doing well up until 2 hours ago when he became acutely agitated, removed his IV, and began yelling loudly. Haloperidol was administered intramuscularly to sedate the patient, and he was resting comfortably on the floor. The patient was found to be unresponsive after the nurse went to check on him due to a telemetry alarm for an HR of 155.

Based on the history, which of the following heart rhythms is the most likely diagnosis?

- A. Atrial fibrillation with rapid ventricular response
- B. Paroxysmal supraventricular tachycardia
- C. Polymorphic ventricular tachycardia with prolonged QT interval
- D. Junctional tachycardia
- E. Monomorphic ventricular tachycardia

515.

After rounds, you return to check on Ms. Todd, an 83-year-old woman recovering from urosepsis. Earlier on rounds, you found that she was pleasant and talkative and even joking with the attending. She seems drowsy, and when you arouse her to examine her, she has difficulty following your commands. She has been in the hospital for 2 weeks awaiting placement for subacute rehab, and no family members have been by to see her this week. The nurse reports that she seems to perk up during rounds and at meals, but that other times during the day, she has difficulty with memory and answering questions.

What is the most likely diagnosis?

- A. Major depressive disorder
- B. Medication side effect
- C. Acute delirium
- D. Early dementia
- E. Normal behavior for elderly inpatient

516.

You are called to evaluate a delirious 73-year-old man admitted for CHF exacerbation complicated by acute renal failure and HAP. His past medical history is significant for longstanding Parkinson disease. He has pulled out his IV for the second time this evening, and has gotten out of bed and yelled at the nurse in front of the nurses' station. They have repeatedly tried to redirect him back to his room without success. You find him standing next to his bed with hospital security and the nurse.

What is the next best step in the management of this patient?

A. Intramuscular haloperidol
B. Oral haloperidol
C. Oral lorazepam
D. Oral quetiapine
E. Oral trazodone

517.

A 65-year-old woman is brought to your clinic by her children because of depression and weight loss since her husband died 6 months ago. She has smoked 2 packs per day for 40 years. She takes propranolol for mild HTN. She answers your questions but seems markedly disinterested.

BP 126/78, HR 70, Ht 5'6", WT 130 lbs
Exam unremarkable
Routine labs and chest radiograph are normal.

Which of the following is the next best step in management?

A. Discontinue the propranolol and start a thiazide diuretic.
B. Check TSH.
C. Order a total body CT scan.
D. Start an SSRI.
E. Refer for grief counseling.

518.

A 55-year-old man presents to the emergency department with a complaint of increasing discomfort and anxiety over the last 24 hours. He describes feeling jittery and restless and was unable to sleep last night. He now reports onset of nausea while waiting in the emergency department. Past medical history includes diabetes mellitus, hypertension, hyperlipidemia, post-traumatic stress disorder, and chronic low back pain. He is a 2-pack-per-day smoker and drinks 3–4 beers/day. He reports that while on his way to the pharmacy to pick up refills of his medications, he was robbed and was unable to purchase any of his prescribed medications. He has been unable to purchase any alcohol or cigarettes since that time. His current medications include aspirin, metformin, simvastatin, diazepam, paroxetine, and oxycodone/acetaminophen.

Physical exam shows a temp of 99.0° F, HR 105, RR 20, and BP 153/92. He is anxious and has difficulty sitting still during the interview. You also notice the patient yawns frequently. Pupils are 7 mm bilaterally, equal, round, and reactive to light. Abdominal exam reveals hyperactive bowel sounds but otherwise unremarkable.

Which of the following is the likely cause of the patient's symptoms?

A. Cocaine withdrawal
B. Benzodiazepine withdrawal
C. Alcohol withdrawal
D. Opiate withdrawal
E. Nicotine withdrawal

519.

An 84-year-old woman is brought to the clinic by her two daughters. They express concern over their mother's driving. She has become lost twice in the last month and has had at least 2 near misses with other vehicles while driving.

As you discuss the considerations for safe driving and the elderly, which of the following is <u>most</u> accurate?

    A. Arthritic disease may be a sufficient reason to restrict driving privileges.
    B. Night driving should be encouraged for seniors to avoid peak traffic times.
    C. In general, senior citizens tend to have the safest driving records.
    D. Restrictions are not necessary if the patient maintains normal mental functions.

520.

You are asked to evaluate a 42-year-old male in a local homeless center, where you volunteer your services. He has an extended history of bipolar disorder and has had relatively good response to lithium therapy in the past; but he suffers from poor compliance, along with bouts of binge alcohol consumption. He was recently discharged from an admission in the local psychiatric unit after an acute flair of his bipolar disorder. He was stabilized during the admission and discharged with therapeutic lithium levels.

His current lithium level is reported as 1.1 mEq/L (0.6–1.3 mEq/L).

Which side effect from this treatment is <u>most</u> likely?

    A. Nephrotoxicity
    B. Elevated TSH
    C. Pancreatitis
    D. Suicide
    E. Parkinson-like symptoms

521.

A 78-year-old woman is admitted with a perforated duodenal ulcer. She has no history of alcohol use. After surgery, she is moved to the ICU. During her ventilator wean, she is extremely confused, does not know where or who she is, and keeps trying to crawl out of bed. She fluctuates between periods of somnolence and wakefulness.

What would be the best way to manage this patient?

    A. 2-point restraints.
    B. 4-point restraints.
    C. Keep a sitter at the bedside.
    D. Treatment with haloperidol.
    E. Treatment with meperidine.

522.

Anorexia nervosa is a serious eating disorder that can lead to life-threatening physiologic compromise. Its underlying psychological component is often very resistant to intervention. Long-term recovery is possible in a portion of affected individuals.

Which of the following is the <u>most</u> common long-term consequence in patients who have recovered from anorexia nervosa?

A. Obesity
B. Reduced bone mass
C. Menstrual abnormalities
D. Thyroid abnormalities
E. Kidney abnormalities

523.

During a routine physical examination with a 32-year-old female, you note fullness over the parotids bilaterally. This area is <u>not</u> tender, and the oral mucosa is unremarkable.

Examination of her teeth, however, reveals discoloration and apparent loss of significant amounts of dental enamel.

On direct questioning, the patient confides that she is concerned about her weight and has been experiencing frequent episodes of vomiting after large meals. She admits to occasionally inducing the emesis to alleviate frequent uncomfortable feelings of satiety.

Which of the following is indicated or documented at this point?

A. Hospitalization to correct underlying disorders and nutrition.
B. Antidepressants, such as fluoxetine.
C. Cognitive behavioral therapy has no useful role in her therapeutic plan.
D. Her disease is genetically based and is evenly distributed worldwide.

524.

A 28-year-old male presents as a new patient. He states that he has adult attention deficit disorder (ADD). He left his previous provider because of disagreements over medication refills. You obtain the following historical information.

The patient did well in school until age 13 when he started experiencing conflicts with authority figures. At that time, he experimented with marijuana and currently uses both marijuana and alcohol on a daily basis. His school performance fell from A's and B's in the 5th grade to C's and D's in the 7th grade. He dropped out of school at the age of 15 years. He has divorced twice and has been unable to keep employment for more than 6 months at a time. He has significant difficulty with sleep and states that he always feels distracted. He states that he has a bad temper and has difficulty controlling his emotions.

Which of the following favors a diagnosis of bipolar disorder (BD) over the diagnosis of attention deficit disorder (ADD)?

A. Active substance abuse
B. Sleep disturbances
C. Poor employment history
D. Emotional outbursts
E. Age of onset

525.

A 20-year-old female presents to the emergency department with a presumed narcotic overdose. You are called in to evaluate her.

You would expect which of the following physical findings:

A. Increased level of consciousness
B. Mydriasis
C. Tachypnea
D. Hypertension
E. Bradycardia

526.

A 38-year-old man presents with a request for "medication for depression." He is a new patient to you, and he has come on advice from his mother, who is your patient. His mother suggested he begin sertraline, a medication you prescribed for her 3 months ago.

He states that his "dot-com" business folded a year ago, and he has been unable to find another job in the computer industry without relocating. He has moved back in with his mother. He describes a fluctuating appetite, anhedonia, and insomnia. He denies weight loss, fever, diarrhea, and skin rashes.

He is single and has a monogamous sexual relationship with his girlfriend.

Which of the following side effects might this patient experience upon prescription of sertraline?

A. Decreased libido
B. Delayed ejaculation
C. Erectile dysfunction
D. Decreased sensation
E. Hypersexuality

527.

You are asked to visit with a 24-year-old female, who was brought to the clinic by her husband. She has been demonstrating extended periods of decreased energy, emotional lability, and lack of pleasure from recreational activities. On further evaluation, you learn that she has had similar experiences since she was 13–14 years old. Her history is also remarkable for several family members with documented long QT interval syndrome. She was evaluated by a cardiologist when she was 19 years old, and now reports that she was told that she had borderline QT interval prolongation.

In discussing treatment options for her depressive symptoms, which of the following poses the greatest risk with her cardiac status?

    A. Selective serotonin reuptake inhibitors (SSRI)
    B. Tricyclic antidepressants (TCA)
    C. Monoamine oxidase inhibitors (MAOI)
    D. Norepinephrine and dopamine reuptake inhibitors (NDRI)

528.

A 30-year-old woman has a 2-year history of irritable mood, hypersomnia, and poor concentration. She reports feeling depressed most of nearly every day. She has never felt manic or had such symptoms.

Which of the following is the <u>most</u> likely diagnosis?

    A. Adjustment disorder
    B. Major depressive disorder
    C. Major depressive episode
    D. Dysthymic disorder
    E. Bipolar disorder

529.

A 36-year-old man presents with complaints of recurrent palpitations and sweating. When these episodes occur, he has "a feeling of doom or dying" and a feeling that he is "not himself"—almost like he is depersonalized. He reports tingling sensations in his fingers and sometimes has trembling. Usually these "episodes" last for 20 minutes. They seem to occur most often when he is about to go out on a date, or he has to visit his mother. Laboratory testing is initiated.

Pending your laboratory testing, what is the <u>most</u> likely diagnosis?

    A. Temporal lobe seizure
    B. Adrenal dysfunction
    C. Vestibular dysfunction
    D. Panic disorder
    E. Pheochromocytoma

530.

A 36-year-old woman comes to you because she has the fear of being in the supermarket when it is crowded. Because of this fear, she goes only at 3 a.m. The symptoms have worsened, including tachycardia, tremor, palpations, sweating, paresthesias, and dizziness. She relates this to an episode that occurred 5 months ago when she was at the supermarket and a fire alarm went off. She was unable to find the exit quickly; ever since, she has been fearful.

What is the most likely diagnosis?

A. Schizophrenia
B. Agoraphobia
C. Drug abuse
D. PVCs
E. Hypoglycemia induced by smelling the bakery

531.

A 38-year-old man presents with 105° F temperature, muscular rigidity, tremor, mental confusion, and diaphoresis. He is unable to communicate and cannot tell you anything about his history.

On physical examination:
   Temperature 105° F, HR 120, BP 160/100, RR 30
   He is confused and unable to communicate. He is diaphoretic.
   He had generalized rigidity (like a "lead pipe").

Which of the following medications would most likely be responsible for his findings?

A. Amitriptyline
B. Lorazepam
C. Haloperidol
D. Bromocriptine
E. Dantrolene

532.

A 45-year-old woman with history of unknown psychiatric disorder presents at the urging of her husband. He says that in the past few months, she has been on a "spending spree." She has always liked to shop, but he says this has gone way over her usual amount. All of their credit cards are "maxed-out," and he has had to take out a home loan to pay some of the bills. He reports that she never seems to sleep and spends hours on the internet buying items or watching the home shopping network and buying things off the television. When you talk with her, she speaks very quickly and seems in a very good mood. He also notes that she is very aggressive sexually and initiates sex frequently, while in the past she had little interest in sex. She also has been telling her husband that the TV talks to her and that it helps her make decisions about what products to buy.

Physical examination is normal.

Which of the following is <u>most</u> likely to be effective in treating her condition?

A. Paroxetine
B. Levothyroxine
C. Thyroid ablation
D. Lithium plus an antipsychotic
E. Lorazepam

533.

A 25-year-old woman is brought in by her husband. He is concerned because she has lost weight and will not eat. The patient admits that she has an intense fear of becoming fat and that she weighs herself 3–4 times a day. She will also cause herself to vomit if she sees she has gained 1/2 pound. She has not had menses in 6 months. You suspect she has anorexia nervosa and refer her for intensive counseling.

Which of the following laboratory abnormalities are you likely to find?

A. Hypercalcemia
B. Hyperkalemia
C. Hypernatremia
D. Hypophosphatemia
E. High TSH

534.

A 40-year-old man with a known history of depression presents for left knee pain. While examining his knee, you ask him how he is doing. He says that lately he has become sadder and sometimes despondent. When you ask him about suicidal thoughts, he says that he has actually thought about killing himself, and he recently bought a gun. He says that he has had suicidal thoughts for about a week. He says that right now he does not feel this way, but this morning before he came to the appointment, he had loaded the gun and had thought about killing himself.

Which of the following is the best management?

A. Immediately admit him by emergency commitment.
B. Because he is not acutely suicidal in your office, discuss with him the need for hospitalization and admit the patient with his consent; if he refuses, set up a follow-up appointment for tomorrow morning.
C. Discuss with him the need for hospitalization and ask him for voluntary admission; if he refuses, then institute emergency commitment.
D. Arrange outpatient follow-up tomorrow morning with a psychiatrist, social worker, and care planner.
E. Increase his antidepressant medication and have him return tomorrow morning.

535.

A mother with bipolar disorder was treated throughout her pregnancy with lithium. She delivers an apparently healthy term female with Apgar scores of 9/9. A holosystolic murmur heard best over the left anterior chest is noted on physical exam.

Which of the following is the <u>most</u> likely diagnosis visible on echocardiography?

A. Enlarged right atrium
B. Atrial septal defect
C. Mitral valve prolapse
D. Ventricular septal defect
E. Aortic stenosis

536.

A 20-year-old female in her third year of college presents with concerns about amenorrhea for 6 months. She also complains of lethargy and a chronic sore throat. Physical exam shows enlargement of the parotid gland and soft palate petechiae.

What would be the <u>most</u> likely abnormality on laboratory testing?

A. Hypercalcemia
B. Hypokalemia
C. Hypernatremia
D. Hyperkalemia
E. Hypoglycemia

537.

An 18-year-old male, recently suspended from school because he threatened several of his peers during a verbal altercation, presents for evaluation to your office. He has had multiple issues in the past with depression and inability to interact with others. His mother states that he has always struggled to make friends, has poor self-esteem, and is frequently teased because he "looks like a girl." Height is at the 90th percentile and weight at the 30th percentile. He is noted to have prominent gynecomastia and small testicles on exam.

Which of the following is the <u>most</u> likely diagnosis?

A. Depression; he should be started on an antidepressant with aggressive appropriate-for-age counseling. Puberty should "kick in" soon.
B. Oppositional defiant disorder made worse by delayed puberty.
C. Bipolar disorder made worse by delayed puberty.
D. Abnormal sex chromosome karyotype results.
E. No pathologic diagnosis; his fertility is normal despite small testicular size.

538.

A 20-year-old female is being evaluated for symptoms of depression associated with frequent mood swings. She is described as an "emotional roller coaster" by her friends and parents. On exam, she has hepatomegaly, and the following concentric circular densities are noted in her cornea:

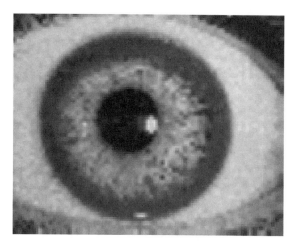

Which of the following tests will confirm the diagnosis?

    A. Alpha-fetoprotein level
    B. Serum haptoglobin level
    C. Total iron-binding capacity
    D. Ceruloplasmin level
    E. Free erythrocyte protoporphyrin

539.

A 25-year-old male is admitted to an inpatient psychiatric unit after a physical altercation with his stepfather. He has a history of violent behavior and depression. Reportedly, he threatened to kill both himself and his stepfather if he was not allowed to drive his stepfather's Mercedes. A urine drug screen is positive for cannabinoids.

Which of the following findings would likely be present on physical examination of this patient?

    A. Gynecomastia
    B. Hepatomegaly
    C. Hypothermia
    D. Bradycardia
    E. Papilledema with associated increased intraocular pressure

MISCELLANEOUS

540.

A 65-year-old man presents with cough and fever. He has had severe diarrhea for 2 days. He was recently on a cruise with a friend who was diagnosed with *Legionella* yesterday.

PMH: diabetes, hyperlipidemia, hypertension
Meds: lisinopril, simvastatin, amlodipine, gemfibrozil, metformin

Chest x-ray shows patchy bilateral infiltrates.
WBC 17,000, Na 125

Which is the <u>most</u> appropriate treatment?

A. Amoxicillin-clavulanate
B. Clarithromycin
C. Levofloxacin
D. Cefuroxime
E. Trimethoprim/sulfamethoxazole

541.

A 38-year-old woman with RA presents with a painful skin lesion that has developed over the past 24 hours. The patient thinks it is a spider bite, but she hasn't seen any spiders. She has had fevers. Meds: prednisone 10 mg qd, hydroxychloroquine 200 mg qd, methotrexate 25 mg/week, omeprazole 20 mg qd, naproxen 500 mg bid.

Which is the <u>most</u> appropriate treatment?

A. Doxycycline
B. TMP/SMX
C. Dicloxacillin
D. Levofloxacin

542.

A new therapy for lung cancer is extremely successful, prolonging life by an average of 3 years. This treatment becomes standard of care for lung cancer patients.

What effect does this have on lung cancer statistics?

A. Increases the incidence
B. Increases the prevalence
C. Increases the sensitivity of screening tests
D. Decreases the specificity of screening tests
E. Reduces the positive predictive value of screening tests

543.

A new blood test is developed to screen for pancreatic cancer. The sensitivity of the test is 75%.

Which of the following is correct?

A. Patients with a negative test result have a 75% chance of not having the disease.
B. Patients with a positive test result have a 75% chance of having the disease.
C. In patients who have the disease, 25% have a negative test result.
D. In patients with a negative test result, 75% do not have the disease.

544.

Which patient would be appropriate to screen for abdominal aortic aneurysm (AAA)?

A. 50-year-old man who presents with chest pain
B. 55-year-old woman who presents with a stroke
C. 60-year-old woman with a 100-pack-year history of smoking
D. 75-year-old woman with a 100-pack-year history of smoking
E. 66-year-old man with a 60-pack-year history of smoking who quit 10 years ago

545.

A 61-year-old man presents to clinic to establish primary care. He is healthy and has no significant medical problems. He has not seen a physician since he had an annual exam at age 50.

Which immunizations would you recommend for him?

A. Annual influenza
B. Annual influenza, Pneumovax®
C. Annual influenza, Tdap, Pneumovax
D. Annual influenza, Tdap, varicella zoster
E. Annual influenza, varicella zoster, Tdap, Pneumovax

546.

A 46-year-old woman with diabetes and seizure disorder presents with nausea and fatigue. Physical exam is unremarkable. Medications: glyburide 5 mg qd, metformin 850 mg bid, phenytoin 300 mg qd, topiramate 400 mg qd, pantoprazole 40 mg qd. Labs: Na 133, K 3.9, Cl 112, HCO_3 13, Glu 158, BUN 18, Cr 1.0.

What is the most likely cause of this patient's acidosis?

A. Phenytoin
B. Topiramate
C. Metformin
D. Pantoprazole

547.

A 55-year-old woman with a history of hypothyroidism presents with increasing fatigue and bradycardia. Her TSH has risen from 4 (a year ago) to 45. Her meds are simvastatin, verapamil, warfarin, citalopram, calcium, and an MVI.

An interaction with which of these is the <u>most</u> likely cause of her increased TSH?

    A. Simvastatin
    B. Verapamil
    C. Warfarin
    D. Citalopram
    E. Calcium

548.

You are seeing a 57-year-old female with osteoporosis (T-1.2 vertebral, T-2.7 femoral neck). Family history of breast cancer in her grandmother at age 58. No other medical problems. Reports three falls in the past year.

Which of the following would you recommend for treatment?

    A. Raloxifene 60 mg PO qd
    B. Ibandronate 150 mg PO q month
    C. Teriparatide 20 mcg SQ daily
    D. Alendronate 70 mg PO q week
    E. No treatment other than calcium and vitamin D

549.

An 84-year-old man presents with hematuria. He had an episode last week, but has had hematuria for the past 4 days. He has had some hesitancy, frequency, and nocturia for several years.

Meds: ASA, MVI, omeprazole

A urinalysis is done that shows RBCs, no WBCs. Cystoscopy shows no bladder malignancy. CT scan of the abdomen shows no renal lesions.

What do you recommend to help prevent future hematuria?

    A. Tamsulosin.
    B. Weekly dose of norfloxacin.
    C. Finasteride.
    D. Pyridium®.
    E. Stop his aspirin.

550.

An 80-year-old Cambodian woman is brought to the emergency department with abdominal pain and nausea. A CT scan is done that shows multiple lesions in the liver and a large pancreatic mass. Her children ask you not to tell her the diagnosis because in their culture it isn't appropriate to inform the patient they have terminal cancer and that they are dying.

What should you do?

    A. Ask the patient if she would like to designate a family member to help make decisions about her care.
    B. Tell the patient that she has cancer and that it is serious.
    C. Tell the patient that she has cancer and that it is terminal.
    D. Tell the family that you have to tell the patient even though they don't want you to.

551.

If the presence of peripheral edema has a sensitivity of 80% and a specificity of 40% for the presence of cirrhosis, what is the positive likelihood ratio if a patient has edema?

    A. 3
    B. 2.4
    C. 2
    D. 1.33
    E. 0.75

552.

If the absence of peripheral pulses has a sensitivity of 90% for PAD and a specificity of 95%, what is the negative likelihood ratio for PAD if a patient has peripheral pulses?

    A. 1.0
    B. 0.5
    C. 0.3
    D. 0.1
    E. 0.05

553.

You are asked to evaluate the usefulness of a new diagnostic test to identify patients with chronic stomach growling syndrome (CSGS). Epidemiologic studies have shown that 1.5% of the population suffers from CSGS. The new test is abnormal in 2.6% of all patients in the same population, and the sensitivity is 98%.

What is the positive predictive value of the new test for CSGS?

A. 98%
B. 77%
C. 57%
D. 43%
E. Cannot be determined from the information given

554.

A 64-year-old man presents with questions about his medications. He was instructed by the pharmacist to talk with his physician regarding potential interactions between his medications and food.

Medical history is significant for gastroesophageal reflux disease, hypertension, hyperlipidemia, depression, and partial androgen deficiency.

Medications:
    Omeprazole 20 mg qd
    Nifedipine XR 60 mg qd
    Hydrochlorothiazide 25 mg qd
    Citalopram 20 mg qd
    Lovastatin 20 mg qhs
    Testosterone injections

From which of the following beverages should this patient abstain?

A. Orange juice
B. Green tea
C. Apple juice
D. Grapefruit juice
E. Lemonade

555.

A national institute looks at whether breastfeeding protects women from developing breast cancer. Six studies are deemed high-quality and are included in the analysis.

The odds ratios (and their 95% confidence intervals [CI]) for each of the studies are:

    0.6 (CI 0.35–1.05)
    0.77 (CI 0.60–1.10)
    0.88 (CI 0.70–1.22)
    0.75 (CI 0.60–1.10)
    0.98 (CI 0.81–1.21)
    0.69 (CI 0.50–1.04)

Based on these 6 studies, which of the following is the **most** accurate conclusion?

A. There is no statistically significant evidence of protection from breastfeeding.
B. There is a small, statistically significant protection from breastfeeding.
C. There is a moderate, statistically significant protection from breastfeeding.
D. There is a small, statistically insignificant increased risk from breastfeeding.
E. There is a small, statistically significant increased risk from breastfeeding.

556.

A 56-year-old man with Type 2 diabetes is hospitalized for treatment of cellulitis. The nursing staff gives 100 units of NPH insulin instead of the ordered 10 units. The mistake is discovered 15 minutes after he received the dose, and you order a dextrose infusion.

What should you tell the patient?

A. He is at risk for low blood sugar because of his infection, so you have prescribed a glucose infusion.
B. A dosage error was made, and he received 10x the insulin dose he was supposed to receive; therefore, he is receiving a glucose infusion to help prevent low blood sugar.
C. He may have too much insulin right now, so he is being put on a glucose infusion to avoid low blood sugar.
D. You are concerned that he could develop low blood sugar today, so you will be monitoring him closely and will prescribe a glucose infusion to prevent low blood sugar.
E. You will discuss this if he inquires about the infusion.

557.

A 57-year-old female with a 22-year history of diabetes mellitus returns for follow-up of persistent right ear pain. She initially presented 5 weeks ago with complaints of right ear pain after attending her water aerobics class and was treated with topical otic gentamicin drops for a 7-day course. She had some slight symptomatic improvement, but the pain persists and is now episodic in nature. She has used the drops intermittently in combination with home remedies of diluted vinegar and hydrogen peroxide.

On examination, the right ear canal demonstrates erythema, swelling, and granulation tissue on the posterior-inferior wall. Neurological exam, particularly of the cranial nerves, is within normal limits. There is tenderness on palpation of the pinna but not over the mastoid process.

Contrast tomography does not reveal osseous abnormalities.

Which of the following is the most appropriate next step in patient care?

A. Biopsy and culture of granulation tissue in the canal
B. Extensive surgical debridement with cultures
C. Empiric antimicrobial coverage for *Pseudomonas*
D. Surface cultures from the external canal
E. Cleansing of the canal and biopsy of granulation tissue

558.

A 25-year-old law school student presents with new-onset hearing loss. She reports that she has had gradual hearing loss for the past 2 weeks. She noted a rash on her extremities, along with a mild fever, about 6 months ago. The rash resolved, and she has been well since; but she has had some persistent lymphadenopathy. She has been sexually active with the same individual for the past 2 years and is monogamous. Neither she nor her boyfriend has had a sexually transmitted disease that she knows of. She lives in Detroit, Michigan, and has no knowledge of tick bites. She has 2 dogs.

Which of the following is the <u>most</u> likely explanation for her hearing loss?

    A. Rubella
    B. Rubeola
    C. Parvovirus B19
    D. *Treponema pallidum*
    E. Early presenile hearing loss

559.

A 63-year-old man presents with complaint of decreased hearing in his right ear. He was recently in the hospital with an *E. coli* bacteremia and received gentamicin and ceftriaxone.

Physical Exam:

HEENT: PERRLA, EOMI
        Ears: Left tympanic membrane normal. Unable to visualize right tympanic membrane due to cerumen.
        Throat: clear
Neuro: Weber test lateralizes to his right ear.
        Rinne test shows air conduction louder in his left ear, bone conduction louder in the right ear.

Which of the following is the <u>most</u> likely cause of his hearing loss?

    A. Gentamicin toxicity
    B. Cerumen impaction
    C. Ménière disease
    D. Acoustic neuroma
    E. Cochlear osteosclerosis

560.

A 75-year-old man who is sexually active has recent onset of impotence. His erections have gradually become inadequate for sexual intercourse. He has chronic stable angina and hypertension. He has taken aspirin and atenolol for more than 20 years.

Which of the following is the <u>most</u> likely cause of his erectile dysfunction?

A. Atenolol
B. Decreased serum testosterone level
C. Vascular disease
D. Neuropathy
E. Normal aging

561.

A 40-year-old woman presents for evaluation of decreased hearing. On Weber testing, the sound lateralizes to the right ear. On Rinne testing of the left ear, the air conduction is the loudest. Hearing testing shows her right ear is normal.

Which of the following is the <u>most</u> likely diagnosis?

A. Excessive cerumen obstructing the left tympanic membrane
B. Left tympanic membrane perforation
C. Acute otitis media
D. Otosclerosis
E. Sensorineural hearing loss of the left ear

562.

A 53-year-old female experienced "white clot syndrome," a severe heparin-induced thrombosis, while receiving prophylactic unfractionated heparin as antithrombotic therapy during a previous hospitalization.

Which of the following is the <u>most</u> appropriate approach to her care?

A. Intravenous heparin poses a significant risk for recurrence, but low-dose subcutaneous heparin may be safely used in the future.
B. Enoxaparin, a low-molecular-weight heparin, should be substituted for prophylaxis in the future.
C. Argatroban should be substituted for subcutaneous heparin in the future.
D. Platelet transfusions should be given immediately to ameliorate the clotting.

563.

A 24-year-old Caucasian college student comes to your office for evaluation of chronic sinus infections. She says that she has had these for "as long as I can remember." She has also always had "trouble with my lungs" and relates incidences that sound like recurrent bronchitis and occasional pneumonia. She now has a thick mucopurulent nasal discharge with sinus tenderness. Also on examination, you note a nasal polyp. You suspect that she has recurrent sinusitis and refer her to an ENT for trans-maxilla sinus culture. This results in a significant growth of *Pseudomonas aeruginosa*.

Which of the following is the <u>most</u> appropriate next step in her management?

    A. Repeat the sinus culture after treating her with ceftriaxone.
    B. Functional endoscopic sinus surgery.
    C. Sweat chloride testing and/or more specific testing for a genetic mutation.
    D. Serum IgE levels.
    E. Nasal smear for eosinophils.

564.

Your front desk calls regarding a 20-year-old male who walked into the clinic with complaints of acute scrotal pain associated with nausea and abdominal pain. He has had similar but less severe symptoms once or twice in the last month; but over the last 5 hours, the pain has become progressively more severe. He has had two new sexual partners over the last 2 months. He does not use condoms.

On examination, he is afebrile. His abdomen is soft with normal bowel sounds. There is no tenderness or rebound. The left testicle is swollen and exquisitely tender with no improvement on scrotal elevation. There is no urethral discharge or other lesions. There is loss of cremasteric reflex on the left side.

Urinalysis is within normal limits.

Which of the following is the <u>most</u> appropriate initial intervention?

    A. Azithromycin orally
    B. Injection of ceftriaxone
    C. Renal ultrasound
    D. Testicular ultrasound
    E. Urine culture

565.

You see a 23-year-old male in the emergency department who presents with confusion and agitation. He spent the previous six hours at a local nightclub where, you have learned through the grapevine, you know multiple drugs are used. The patient has previously been charged with possession of methamphetamine (crystal meth).

Which of the following is <u>most</u> commonly associated with methamphetamine usage?

    A. HIV infection
    B. Hypotension
    C. Hypothermia
    D. Priapism

566.

You are called by nursing staff concerning a 66-year-old female who was admitted 2 days prior for an exacerbation of her COPD. She has an 80-pack-year smoking history and currently smokes 2 packs/day. She has a 10–15-year history of respiratory compromise, and her COPD is becoming increasingly difficult to control with conventional medication regimens. She has demanded several times this morning to be discharged and is now threatening to sign out against medical advice (AMA).

You start your morning rounds with this patient. She continues to have significant respiratory difficulty and is requiring constant O_2 by nasal canula and nebulizer treatments every 2–3 hours. She is also receiving IV antibiotics and steroids. As you try to explain that she is not stable for discharge, she again demands to go home.

Which of the following is the <u>most</u> appropriate next step?

A. Allow the patient to sign herself out AMA.
B. Obtain a stat psychiatry consult.
C. Order a one-time dose of IM haloperidol.
D. Order soft restraints for the patient and continue current therapies.
E. Discuss the use of transdermal nicotine patches with the patient.

567.

A 30-year-old female patient comes to your office and complains that she has been sexually harassed by one of your partners.

What do you recommend?

A. Tell her to obtain an attorney.
B. Ask your partner to explain his actions to her.
C. Have her discuss the issue with your risk-management administrator.
D. Inform the patient that she can no longer be seen in your office and must seek care elsewhere on her own.
E. Refer her to the local medical board.

568.

You see an 80-year-old widowed woman with a history of diabetes mellitus and coronary artery disease after she has suffered her 3rd myocardial infarction in 2 months. She has now had a stroke, and she is paralyzed on her left side and unarousable. CT of the brain shows that the right hemisphere of her brain is almost completely infarcted. She previously indicated to you, and you have documented in your notes, that she does not want to receive artificial life support, including tube feedings, as in the current case of severe debilitation. Her 2 daughters live with her and say they want everything done, including tube feedings. She has no designated power of attorney for medical affairs, and the 2 daughters are "next-in-line" for making medical decisions in your state.

Which of the following is the <u>most</u> appropriate management?

   A. Insist that the tube feedings be continued until the patient can regain capacity and speak for herself.
   B. Tell the daughters that you will ask a court to mediate this decision.
   C. Request an ethics consult.
   D. Discontinue the tube feedings because this is what the patient has informed you as her wish.
   E. Follow the daughters' wishes because they are "next-in-line" for making medical decisions.

569.

A 21-year-old deaf male presents to the emergency room after he "fell out and lost consciousness" during an intramural soccer game. He recovered within "a minute or so." He is alert, oriented, and has a normal physical exam. The patient's brother, who is also deaf, had a similar episode associated with exercise during the previous year.

What is the <u>most</u> likely finding on electrocardiogram?

   A. 2nd degree AV block: Mobitz type 1 (Wenckebach)
   B. Delta wave
   C. Wandering atrial pacemaker
   D. Prolonged QT interval
   E. ST-segment depression

570.

A 21-year-old man presents with fever, irritability, and drooling. He complains of pain when attempting to move his neck and attempts to maintain it in a hyperextended position. Intermittent stridor is noted. He reports that his throat has hurt since falling 3 days ago while running with a stick in his mouth at a fraternity party.

Which of the following is the <u>most</u> likely diagnostic finding in the patient?

   A. A swollen epiglottis on lateral roentgenogram
   B. Increased width of the retropharyngeal space with an air-fluid level on lateral roentgenogram
   C. Asymmetric tonsillar bulge with deviation of the uvula on examination of the oropharynx
   D. Gingival edema associated with a displaced tooth on examination of the oropharynx
   E. A foreign body on lateral roentgenogram

571.

A 53-year-old resident of a long-term mental health facility presents with chronic cough and nasal discharge that he has had for 2 months. He has had only marginal response to 2 courses of antibiotics. Physical exam is positive for bilateral nasal drainage that is noticeably more profuse from the left side of the nose, as well as for dark purple-red circles beneath the eyes. A foul odor is noted during the exam.

What is the <u>most</u> likely diagnosis?

A. Chronic sinusitis
B. Nasal polyp
C. Nasal foreign body
D. Allergic rhinitis
E. Cough variant asthma

572.

Pertussis is on the rise in the United States, and adults are now recognized to be at increased risk. Thus, immunization of all adults is now recommended.

Which of the following is accurate when reviewing the epidemiology of pertussis?

A. Patients with pertussis often have elevated WBC counts with a predominance of neutrophils.
B. The patient is most infectious during the paroxysmal stage of pertussis.
C. The catarrhal stage of pertussis is difficult to clinically distinguish from an otherwise uncomplicated upper respiratory infection.
D. Pertussis is exceedingly rare in adolescents who were fully immunized (i.e., received five doses of pertussis containing vaccine by 6 years of age).

573.

A 28-year-old female presents with a severe sore throat.

Which of the following associated findings are <u>most</u> suggestive of group A streptococcal (GAS) disease?

A. A lack of associated upper respiratory findings and complaints
B. The presence of tender posterior cervical and postauricular lymphadenopathy
C. Presentation during the late spring and summer months
D. Hepatosplenomegaly on abdominal exam
E. An urticarial rash most prominent on the trunk

574.

A 30-year-old man presents tearfully and claims that he tried to commit suicide by taking a bunch of pills in his household. He won't tell you what he took but says it is an over-the-counter medication. You suspect that he may have taken aspirin based on his clinical findings and laboratory data.

Which of the following constellation of symptoms and signs is <u>most</u> consistent with salicylate poisoning?

A. Nausea, vomiting, and pallor followed by jaundice and hepatic failure within 72 hours
B. Coma, seizures, increased respiratory rate, and a "bitter almond" odor
C. Development of intestinal strictures several months after the overdose
D. Increased respiratory rate, fever, lethargy progressing to coma, diaphoresis, and early alkalosis followed by acidosis
E. Delirium, increased heart rate, fever, dry skin and mouth, and urinary retention

APPENDIX A
REFERENCE COLOR PHOTOS

Figure 1, Pulmonary Medicine, Question 52

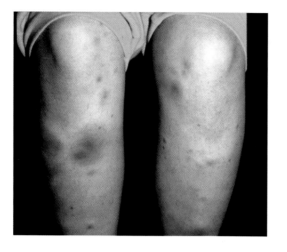

Figure 4, Infectious Disease, Question 199

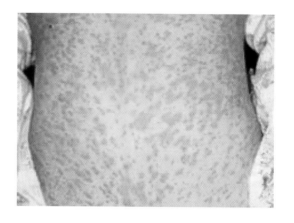

Figure 2, Cardiology, Question 107

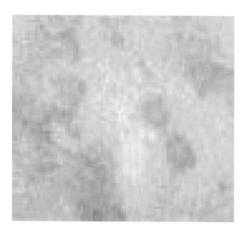

Figure 5, Infectious Disease, Question 200

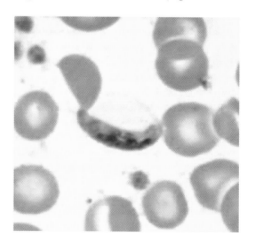

Figure 3, Infectious Disease, Question 192a

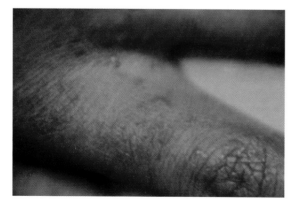

Figure 6, Infectious Disease, Question 205

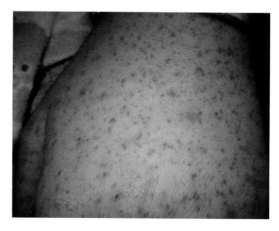

Figure 7, Infectious Disease, Question 206

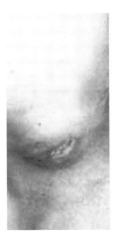

Figure 10, Infectious Disease, Question 216

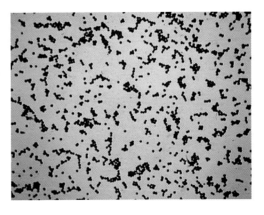

Figure 8, Infectious Disease, Question 213

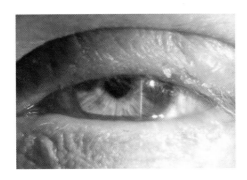

Figure 11, Infectious Disease, Question 223

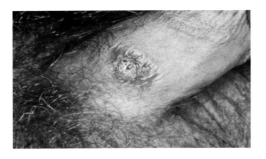

Figure 12, Infectious Disease, Question 225

Figure 9, Infectious Disease, Question 215

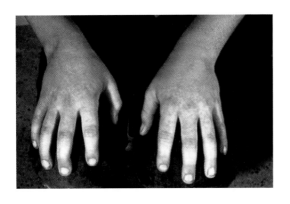

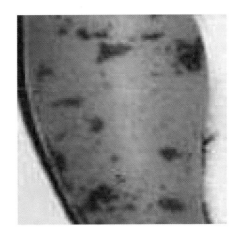

Figure 13, Infectious Disease, Question 227

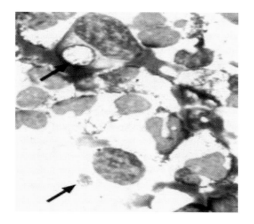

Figure 16, Hematology, Question 330

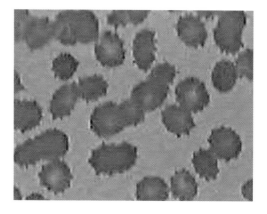

Figure 14, Hematology, Question 328

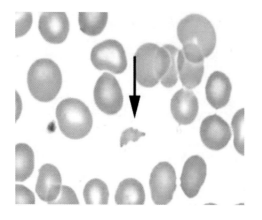

Figure 17, Hematology, Question 331

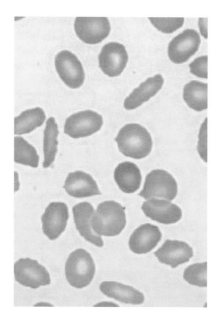

Figure 15, Hematology, Question 329

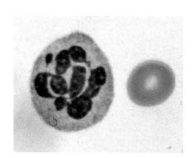

Figure 18, Hematology, Question 332

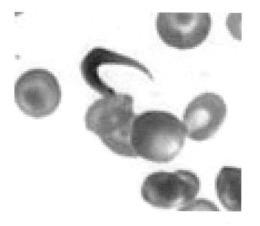

Figure 19, Hematology, Question 333

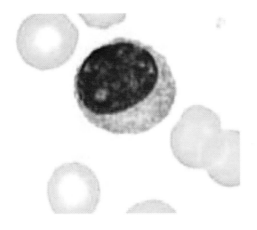

Figure 22, Hematology, Question 336

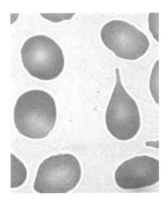

Figure 20, Hematology, Question 334

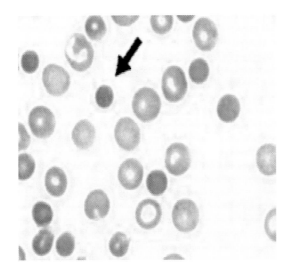

Figure 23, Oncology, Question 369

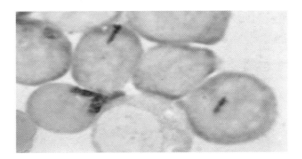

Figure 24, Rheumatology, Question 419

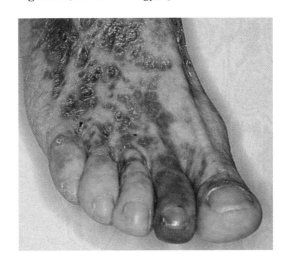

Figure 21, Hematology, Question 335

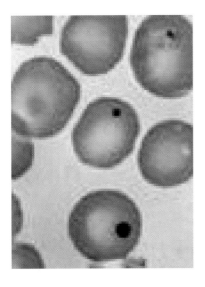

Figure 25, Rheumatology, Question 436

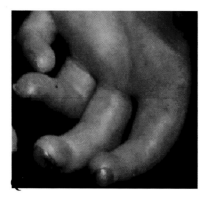

Figure 26, Rheumatology, Question 438

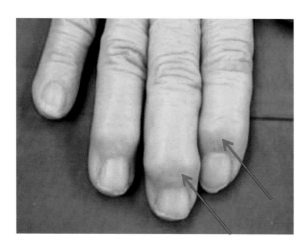

Figure 27, Dermatology, Question 469

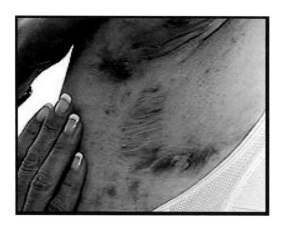

Figure 28, Dermatology, Question 471a

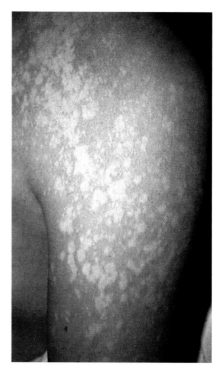

Figure 29, Dermatology, Question 471b

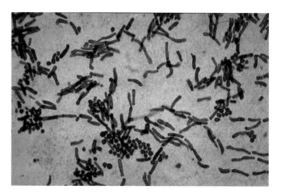

Figure 30, Dermatology, Question 476

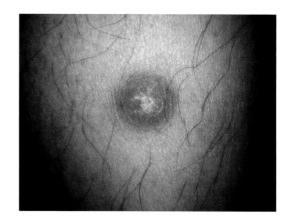

Figure 31, Dermatology, Question 479

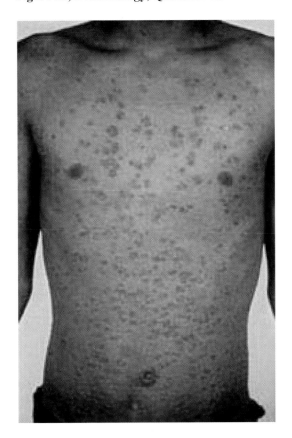

Figure 33, Dermatology, Question 484

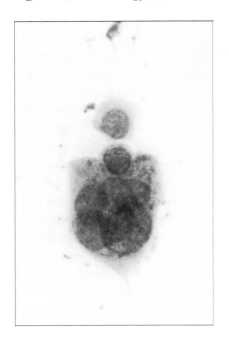

Figure 34, Dermatology, Question 485

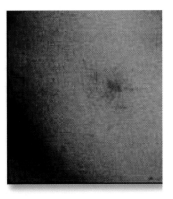

Figure 32, Dermatology, Question 480

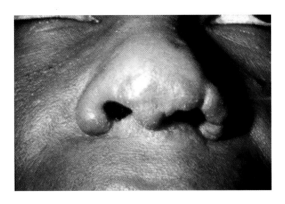

Figure 35, Ophthalmology, Question 505

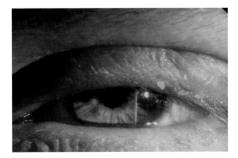

Figure 36, Ophthalmology, Question 512

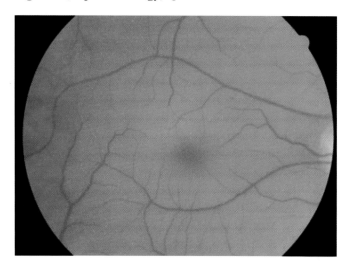

Figure 37, Psychiatry, Question 538

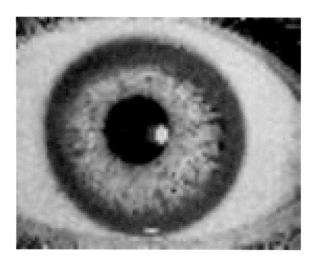

APPENDIX B
NORMAL LABORATORY VALUES

NORMAL LABORATORY VALUES

Blood, Plasma, Serum	Reference Range	SI Reference Intervals
Alanine aminotransferase (ALT, SGPT)	0–0.58 μkat/L	0–35 U/L
Amylase, serum	60–160 Somogyi units/dL	60–180 U/L
Aspartate aminotransferase (AST, SGOT)	0–0.58 μkat/L	0–35 U/L
Bilirubin, serum (adult) Total // Direct	0.1–1.0 mg/dL // 0.0–0.3 mg/dL	2–17 μmol/L // 0–5 μmol/L
Calcium, serum	8.4–11 mg/dL	2.1–2.8 mmol/L
Cholesterol, serum-desirable	< 200 mg/dL	< 5.2 mmol/L
Cholesterol, serum-borderline	200–239 mg/dL	5.2–6.18 mmol/L
Cholesterol, serum-undesirable	> 240 mg/dL	> 6.2 mmol/L
Creatine kinase, serum (total)	Male: 55–170 U/L	55–170 U/L
	Female: 30–135 U/L	30–106 U/L
Creatinine, serum	0.6–1.2 mg/dL	53–106 μmol/L
Electrolytes, serum		
Sodium	135–147 mEq/L	135–147 mmol/L
Chloride	95–105 mEq/L	95–105 mmol/L
Potassium	3.5–5.0 mEq/L	3.5–5.0 mmol/L
Bicarbonate	22–28 mEq/L	22–28 mmol/L
Ferritin, serum	Male: 15–200 ng/mL	15–200 μg/L
	Female: 12–150 ng/mL	12–150 μg/L
Gases, arterial (room air)		
pO_2	80–100 mmHg	11.0–13.0 kPa
pCO_2	34–45 mmHg	4.4–5.9 kPa
pH	7.35–7.45	7.35–7.45
Glucose, serum	Fasting: 70–110 mg/dL 2 hr postprandial < 120mg/dL	3.8–6.1 mmol/L < 6.6 mmol/L
Growth Hormone, serum	Fasting: < 5 ng/ml Provocative stimuli: > 7μg/mL	< 5 μg/L > 7 μg/L
Immunoglobulins, serum		
IgA	76–390 mg/dL	0.76–3.90 g/L
IgE	0–380 IU/mL	0–380 μg/L
IgG	650–1,500 mg/dL	6.5–15 g/L
IgM	40–345 mg/dL	0–3.45 g/L

Iron	50–170 μg/dL	9–30 μmol/L
Lactate dehydrogenase	60–120 μkat/L	35–88 U/L
Osmolality, serum	275–295 mOsmol/kg	275–295 mOsmol/kg
Parathyroid hormone, serum, N-terminal	230–630 pg/mL	230–630 ng/L
Phosphatase (alkaline), serum	30–120 U/L	0.5–2 nkat/L
Phosphorus (inorganic), serum	3.0–4.5 mg/dL	1.0–1.4 mmol/L
Prolactin, serum	< 20 ng/mL	< 20 μg/L
Proteins, serum		
— Total (recumbent)	6.0–7.8 g/dL	60–78 g/L
— Albumin	3.5–5.5 g/dL	35–55 g/L
— Globulins	2.3–3.5 g/dL	23–35 g/L
Thyroid stimulating hormone, serum/plasma	2–10 μU/mL	2–10 mU/L
Thyroidal (radioactive) iodine uptake	6–30% of administered dose/ 24 hr	0.06–0.30/24 hr
Thyroxine (T_4), serum	5–12 μg/dL	64–155 mmol/L
Triglycerides, serum	35–160 mg/dL	0.4–1.81mmol/L
Urea nitrogen, serum (BUN)	7–18 mg/dL	1.2–3 mmol/L
Uric acid, serum	3.0–8.2 mg/dL	0.18–0.48 mmol/L

Cerebrospinal Fluid	**Reference Range**	**SI Reference Intervals**
Cell count	0–5 cells/mm^3	0–5 X 106/L
Glucose	40–70 mg/dL	2.2–3.9 mmol/L
Pressure	70–180 mmH$_2$O	70–180 mmH$_2$O
Proteins, total	< 40 mg/dL	< 0.40 g/L

Hematologic	Reference Range	SI Reference Intervals
Bleeding time (template)	2–7 minutes	2–7 minutes
Erythrocyte count	Male: 4.3–5.9 x 10^6/mm^3 Female: 3.5–5.5 x 10^6/mm^3	4.3–5.9 x 10^{12}/L 3.5–5.5 x 10^{12}/L
Hematocrit	Male: 41–53% Female: 36–46%	0.41–0.53 0.36–0.46
Hemoglobin, blood	Male: 13.5–17.5 g/dL Female: 12.0–16.0 g/dL	2.09–2.71 mmol/L 1.86–2.48 mmol/L
Hemoglobin, plasma	1–4 mg/dL	0.16–0.62 μmol/L
Leukocyte count and differential		
Leukocyte count	4,500–11,000/mm^3	4.5–11 x 10^6/L
Segmented neutrophils	54–62%	0.54–0.62
Band forms	3–5%	0.03–0.05
Eosinophils	1–3%	0.01–0.03
Basophils	0–0.75%	0–0.0075
Lymphocytes	25–33%	0.25–0.33
Monocytes	3–7%	0.03–0.07
Mean corpuscular hemoglobin	25.4–34.6 pg/cell	0.39–0.54 fmol/L
Mean corpuscular hemoglobin concentration	31–36% g Hb/cell	4.81–5.58 mmol g Hb/L
Mean corpuscular volume	86–98 μm^3 ~80 - 100	86–98 fl
Partial thromboplastin time	Comparable to control	Comparable to control
Platelet count	150,000–400,000/mm^3	150–400 x 10^9/L
Prothrombin time	< 2 sec deviation from control	< 2 sec deviation from control

Red Cell Distribution Width RDW 11.5 – 14.5